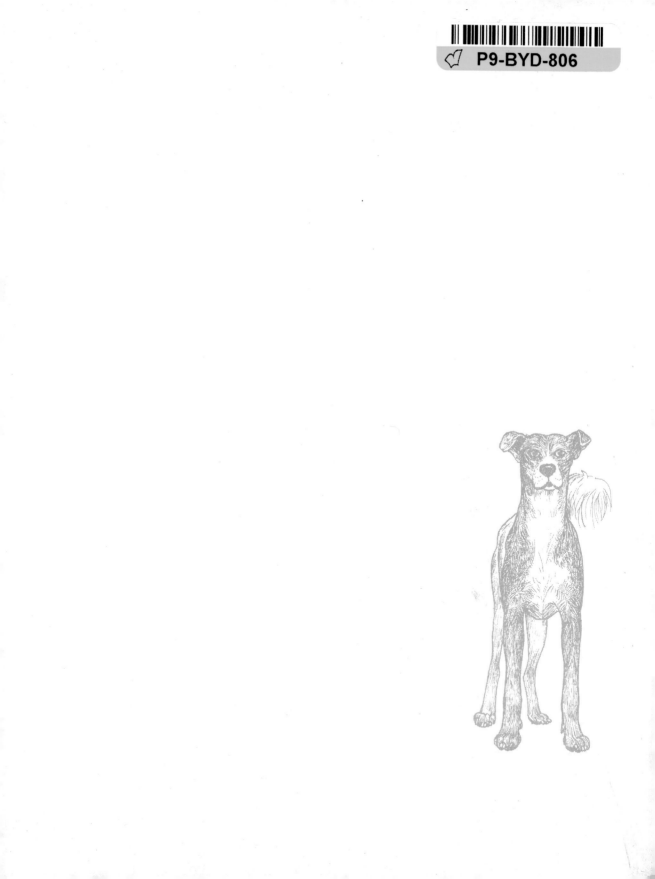

The Veterinarians' Guide to Your Dog's Symptoms

Michael S. Garvey, D.V.M.

Ann E. Hohenhaus, D.V.M.

Katherine A. Houpt, V.M.D., Ph.D.

John E. Pinckney, D.V.M.

Melissa S. Wallace, D.V.M.

Elizabeth Randolph

VILLARD · NEW YORK

The
Veterinarians' Guide
to Your
Dog's Symptoms

Library of Congress Cataloging-in-Publication Data

The veterinarians' guide to your dog's symptoms / Michael S. Garvey . . . [et al.].
      p. cm.
      Includes index.
      ISBN 0-375-75226-9
        1. Dogs—Diseases—Diagnosis. 2. Symptoms in animals.
      I. Garvey, Michael S.
      SF991.V43 1999
      636.7'089—dc21   98-39150

Random House website address: www.atrandom.com

Printed in the United States of America on acid-free paper

9 8 7 6 5 4 3 2

DESIGNED BY BARBARA MARKS

This book is in no way meant to take the place of the medical advice of a veterinarian. A pet owner should consult a veterinarian regularly about the health of his or her dog, in particular if the animal shows any signs/symptoms of illness. The signs/symptoms listed in this book, and the medical conditions they may indicate, are in no way intended to be all-inclusive. They are merely the most commonly seen signs/symptoms in the clinical experiences of the contributing veterinarians.

For Daisy.

May she lead

a long and

healthy life.

Acknowledgments

Thanks to Mollie Doyle at Villard for her patience, calm, and understanding; to Annik LaFarge; and to Barbara Lowenstein, without whom this project would never have happened. Thanks in particular to Norman Kurz at Lowenstein Associates for his help.

Thanks also to Drs. Michael Garvey, Ann Hohenhaus, Katherine Houpt, and Melissa Wallace for their contributions, and especially to Dr. John Pinckney for his heroic efforts.

Last, but by no means least, thanks to my husband, Arthur Hettich, for his continuing encouragement and support.

—Elizabeth Randolph

Contents

Charts and Tables

Illustrations

A Note to the Reader

There are many books on the market designed to assist people in understanding their bodies and health. Several are based on symptoms of disease so that a person can find his symptoms and discover what the most common medical causes of these symptoms may be. There has not been a similar book for pet owners until now. The authors have written this book to help pet owners recognize the medical causes of problems with their dogs and the appropriate steps to take.

One of the difficulties in writing about medical topics for a nonmedical audience is terminology. Words have very specific meanings and are used very carefully in medicine. Many unfamiliar medical terms will be used in this book, and because the intended audience is nonmedical, we have included a glossary at the back of this book.

Among the terminology problems is the fact that the words *symptom* and *sign* are both used in this book. By definition, a *symptom* is a human patient's subjective observation of various pieces of evidence that something may be wrong, which he is able to communicate to his doctor. A *sign* is something that is objectively seen, felt, smelled, or heard. Because a dog cannot communicate her physical feelings except in the most general way (i.e., change in behavior), she technically cannot have symptoms, and an owner or veterinarian must look for signs of medical trouble. However, because most people are familiar with the use of the word *symptom* rather than *sign,* we have used both terms interchangeably in this book.

—Michael S. Garvey, D.V.M.

The
Veterinarians' Guide
to Your
Dog's Symptoms

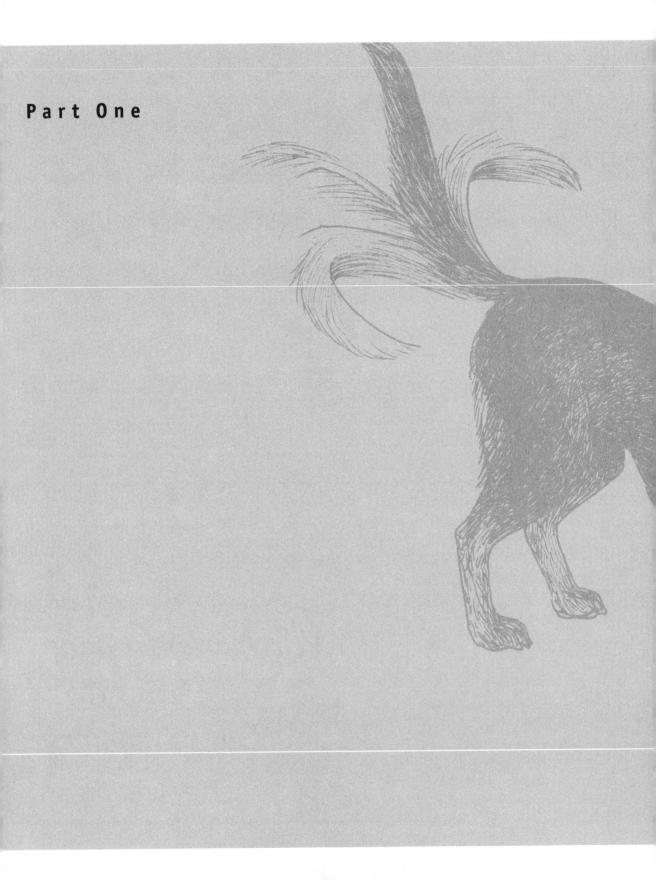

Part One

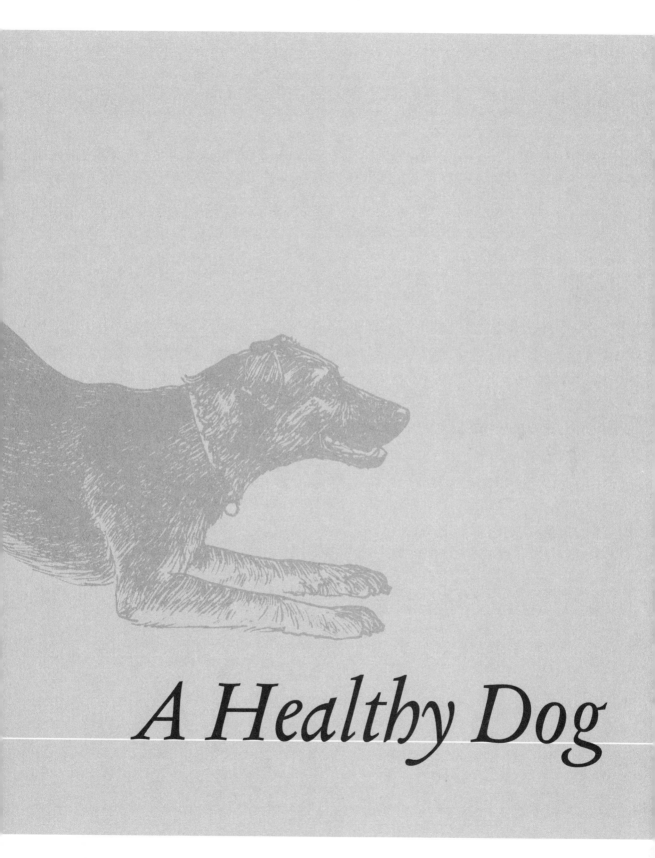

A Healthy Dog

A Healthy

Dog's Body

This chapter contains short descriptions of the various systems in the bodies of normal, healthy dogs, touching on the differences between dogs and humans and between dog body types and breeds. The primary purpose of the chapter is to provide dog owners with a basis of comparison in case a dog's body seems not to be functioning correctly.

In general, dogs' bodies work in much the same way as those of all other mammals, humans included. And although dogs may differ greatly in size, type of haircoat, nose and ear shape, and length of tail, they are all alike physiologically: a 6-pound Yorkshire terrier has all of the same parts as a 150-pound Newfoundland.

Some of the external differences in dogs' bodies, such as eye and facial shape, length of coat, and ear type, may indicate susceptibilities to specific problems.

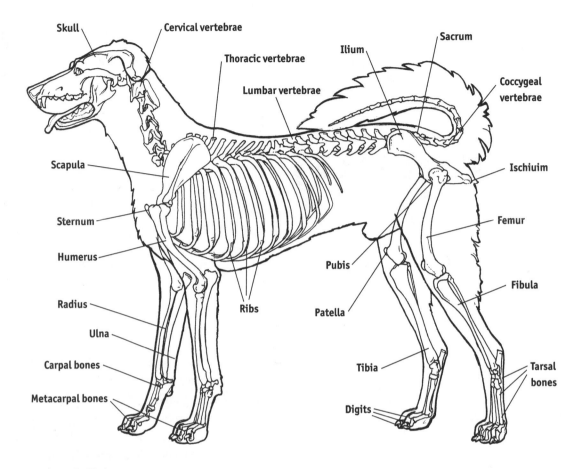

Skull
Cervical vertebrae
Thoracic vertebrae
Ilium
Sacrum
Lumbar vertebrae
Coccygeal vertebrae
Scapula
Ischiuim
Sternum
Femur
Humerus
Pubis
Radius
Fibula
Ribs
Patella
Ulna
Carpal bones
Tibia
Tarsal bones
Metacarpal bones
Digits

A Normal Dog's Skeleton

Skin and Hair

One of the most immediately recognized differences in dogs is the type and length of their hair, or coat. A dog's coat forms an insulating layer between his skin and the external environment. It helps to keep him warm in winter and protects him from the heat and sun in summer. A dog's coat can be short, medium, or long and is either coarse or fine. German shepherds' short, coarse coats are the standard for "normal," because they are most like the coats of coyotes and wolves. Many dogs have what is called a "double coat," consisting of two layers of hair: a downy undercoat and longer, coarser, outercoat. Different types of coats require specific kinds of care and grooming.

All dogs lose hair, or shed, all year long. Dogs with double coats may shed large amounts of fur from their undercoats in the spring and fall. This is known as "blowing" the coat. Although all dogs should be groomed regularly, it is especially important to groom long-coated dogs often or the shed hairs will form mats and tangles instead of falling out.

Dogs' skin plays many important roles. Not

only does it protect a dog's body from the loss of fluids, electrolytes, and proteins, but it also serves as a barrier against infection. Unlike humans, dogs do not perspire through their skin to cool themselves, but only through their feet. This is an inefficient cooling system because the surface area for evaporation is very small. Therefore, dogs also help to cool themselves by panting, which allows water evaporation from the tongue and mouth. In some cases excess panting may be a sign of disease.

Their skin also helps maintain body temperature. The blood vessels in the skin either dilate to cool the body, or constrict to retain body heat when it's cold. A dog's skin also performs the same function as human skin: it conveys sensations of touch, pain, heat, cold, and so on.

A healthy dog's coat is shiny and full and his skin is clear and free of sores, scabs, redness, or scaly patches. A scruffy-looking coat or dry skin can be signs of a dermatologic problem or may indicate a systemic illness. If dark brown or black spots are present on a dog's skin from the time of birth, they may be normal pigmentation, but if spots or discoloration should suddenly appear, they should be examined by a veterinarian for diagnosis.

Eyes and Vision

Although dogs' eyes have the same parts as humans', they differ in their makeup. Dogs' eyes have more rods than human eyes do, which means dogs have much better vision in dim light than do people. On the other hand, human eyes contain more cones than do dogs', enabling people to perceive and differentiate color better. Dogs do, however, see some colors and are not completely color-blind, as was once believed.

Owners are sometimes concerned when a dog's eyes seem to have a bluish or yellowish glare when the animal is looking toward the light. This is the reflection from a region of the retina called the tapetum. The tapetum reflects light back to the retina, further enhancing a dog's night vision. Dogs over eight years of age sometimes develop a cloudy appearance to the lenses of their eyes. This condition may be nuclear (lenticular) sclerosis (see page 111), which does not affect a dog's vision, but should be distinguished from cataracts by a veterinarian.

Another possible cause for owner concern is a pinkish membrane that sometimes appears in the inside corner of a dog's eye, partially covering the eyeball. This membrane is called a third eyelid (nictating membrane) and is present in all mammals except humans. The third eyelid pops up automatically when a dog retracts its eyes (pulls them back into the eye sockets). It protects and cleans the eyeball and is more noticeable in dogs with prominent eyes and flat faces (brachycephalic breeds) such as pugs, Pekingese, Boston terriers, English bulldogs, and Lhasa apsos. Because their eyes are not set deep into their sockets, these dogs are very susceptible to eye damage. A common eye condition in some dogs is cherry eye, in which the glands in the third eyelid become enlarged and appear like a red cherry in the corner of the eye (see page 111).

Sight hounds, or coursing dogs such as greyhounds, Afghans, borzois, Irish wolfhounds, salukis, and Scottish deerhounds, locate and chase their prey by sight rather than scent. They have been selectively bred to have a highly developed sense of sight that is particularly sensitive to motion.

Ears and Hearing

Dogs' internal ears have the same parts as human ears. The outer ear, called the pinna, may be upright (perked) or pendulous and floppy. Dogs with floppy ears are more likely than those with perked ears to develop ear infections, especially if their ears are hairy. The pendulous pinnae of basset hounds, retrievers, all types of spaniels, Irish setters, and poodles, for example, prevent proper air circulation and the hair may plug the opening of the ear. Floppy-eared dogs also frequently suffer from damage to their ear flaps. Dogs with upright ears are more prone to attack by biting flies in the spring and summer if they spend a lot of time outdoors.

Dogs' sense of hearing has evolved over the years to be very acute. Next to smell it is their most highly developed sense and has been estimated to be over 100 percent keener than humans'. They can seemingly differentiate between sound frequencies better than humans and are able to hear much higher-pitched sounds. They can also pinpoint exactly where a sound is coming from.

Noses and a Sense of Smell

Dog noses come in three basic shapes: long and pointy (e.g., collie), normal (e.g., retriever), or brachycephalic (e.g., pug). Brachycephalic breeds are more prone to nasal disorders, may snore, and often have a difficult time breathing when it is extremely hot and humid.

No matter what the shape of their noses, all dogs have an exceptionally acute sense of smell. It is estimated that their olfactory sense is close to one hundred times keener than that of humans.

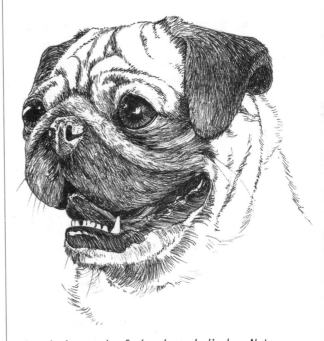

A typical example of a brachycephalic dog. Note the protuberant, exposed eyeballs, extremely short pushed-in nose, and small nostrils.

This is because the olfactory (smell sensing) areas of dogs' brains are much bigger and more highly developed than peoples'. Some breeds, such as the bloodhound, have been bred over the years to be able to identify and isolate specific odors. Because of their very highly developed sense of smell, hunting dogs such as retrievers and beagles are often utilized by various law enforcement agencies to detect bombs, drugs, and even illegally imported fruits and vegetables. Search-and-rescue dogs can even detect a human body submerged in water.

Mouth and Teeth

Dogs' teeth serve two purposes. They can be used as weapons if necessary, but the primary purpose of teeth in domesticated dogs is for eating. Because dogs do not chew their food before swallowing as humans do, but gulp it down, their teeth are designed to tear food into bits suitable for gulping.

Puppies have a total of twenty-eight teeth, evenly divided between the lower and upper jaws. By the time a pup is six to seven months old, his baby teeth will have been replaced by a full set of forty-two adult teeth. During this seven-month period teething may be difficult for a puppy and he may chew excessively. Even long after a puppy's permanent teeth have erupted he may continue to chew a great deal for up to two or more years of age. Owners should be sure to provide teething pups and young adult dogs with suitable chew toys.

Cardiovascular System

The cardiovascular system of dogs is very similar to that of humans. Dogs have a four-chambered *heart* with two atria and two ventricles. The heart is primarily responsible for the pumping and circulation of blood through an elaborate network of *arteries,* which deliver oxygenated blood to tissues, and *veins,* which drain deoxygenated blood from tissues and return it to the heart. Blood is then pumped to the lungs for reoxygenation during respiration.

In general, dogs do not suffer from the types of cardiovascular diseases that humans do. For example, arteriosclerosis, or plaques on the inside of arteries caused by an excess of cholesterol, is virtually unheard of in dogs. Unlike humans, dogs almost never suffer from heart attacks brought about by clogged arteries. Dogs do have other types of heart problems, however, which will be discussed later.

Digestive System

A dog's digestive system prepares food for absorption and distributes it, along with water and other nutrients, to the animal's body. The digestive system is particularly important in maintaining the proper balance of water, electrolytes, minerals, vitamins, and nutrients. The digestion of food releases nutrients such as amino acids, sugars, and other things needed for energy so that the body can also eliminate those parts of food it has not yet digested or utilized.

The beginning of the digestive system is the *esophagus,* a long, muscular tube that runs from the back of the throat to the stomach. Food that is swallowed in pieces is propelled from the throat down the esophagus to the *stomach.* The stomach then grinds and churns the food with acid and some enzymes and prepares the food for the process of digestion. As the digested food leaves the stomach it enters the *small intestine,* where it is further broken down and turned into small, usable particles that are absorbed into the bloodstream and carried to the appropriate parts of the body. This process is helped with enzymes from the *pancreas* and bile from the *liver.*

The liver is a very important and complex organ, responsible for a tremendous number of functions, including the manufacture of proteins, which a dog's body needs in order to perform a myriad of tasks, among them the ability to have normal blood clotting. The liver stores sugars for use to provide energy between meals. It also metabolizes and detoxifies a variety of substances that are ingested or in other ways enter the body, including most drugs, pharmaceuticals, poisons, and chemicals, which are then excreted from a dog's body in bile or urine.

The small intestine ends in the *colon* or *large*

intestine, which functions mainly to continue the process of absorption. A lot of water from food is absorbed in the colon, which is then responsible for propelling waste products out of the dog's body through the *rectum* and *anus.*

Endocrine System

Many *glands,* found in many different locations in a dog's body, make up the endocrine system. Endocrine glands make *hormones* and secrete them into an animal's bloodstream. The hormones are then responsible for attaching themselves to receptors in other organs, thereby allowing necessary functions to occur.

Some of the endocrine glands that are important are the *thyroid glands,* which exert a major impact on an animal's metabolism and regulate how rapidly the body's metabolic functions occur. The *parathyroid glands,* located near the thyroid glands, are important in regulating the level of calcium and phosphorus in the bloodstream. *Adrenal glands,* which are near the *kidneys,* secrete a variety of important hormones, such as cortisol and other hormones that regulate blood pressure and electrolyte balance.

Part of the endocrine system also includes a network of cells in the *pancreas* that secrete insulin and other hormones that help utilize and assimilate sugars and other nutrients.

There are also a variety of *reproductive hormones* that the glands secrete. The ovaries and pituitary glands are responsible for normal heat cycles, egg production, and uterine health in female dogs. The testicles produce hormones responsible for male sexual characteristics and behavior, and normal sperm production.

If a particular endocrine organ oversecretes or undersecretes hormones, diseases occur in a dog's body; this will be discussed later on in this book.

Musculoskeletal System

A dog's musculoskeletal system contains most of the same parts as those of humans, except dogs have no clavicles (collarbones). Because a dog walks on all fours instead of upright, the front legs carry half of his body weight and are very well developed.

Nervous System

Just as in humans, a dog's nervous system is basically broken up into two different areas, the *central nervous system* and the *peripheral nervous system.* The central nervous system includes the *brain* and the *spinal cord,* which runs from the back of the brain through small bones or vertebrae in the spine along almost the entire length of a dog's body.

The brain is responsible for thinking, memory, and cognitive function. The spinal cord accepts impulses from peripheral sensory nerves located everywhere on a dog's body, especially the legs and feet, and brings important information to the brain such as sensations of cold, heat, pain, and touch. It is also responsible for relaying messages from the brain to the rest of the body via the peripheral nerves.

The peripheral nervous system includes the twelve cranial nerves that come out of the brain and are responsible for all of the things that occur from the neck up, including vision, smell, and hearing. Peripheral nerves that branch out of the brain and the spinal cord also transmit messages to the muscles, telling them either to contract or relax so the dog can stand, walk, and move normally. These are called *motor nerves.* Other peripheral nerves carry impulses to the spinal cord. These nerves "sense" cold, heat, pressure, and so forth, and are called *sensory nerves.*

Reproductive System

The reproductive systems of dogs have the same components as those of all other mammals.

Depending on breed and size, dogs reach puberty at anywhere from six to twelve months, and are sexually mature two to three months afterward. Small breeds develop faster, while giant breeds such as Great Danes, Newfoundlands, and Irish wolfhounds are often not sexually mature until over a year of age.

The female *heat cycle* usually occurs twice a year: signs of heat include a swelling of the external genitalia (vulva) and a red to pink discharge from the vulva. Many female dogs keep themselves so clean it can be difficult for an owner to tell when they're in heat. Frequently a gathering of ardent male dogs around the house, or avidly attentive males when the dog is outside, are the first signs to an owner that a heat cycle has begun. To prevent accidental breeding and pregnancy, a female dog in heat must be confined for at *least* twenty-one days from the onset of the heat period, or until *all* signs of heat are completely gone.

Female dogs have five *mammary glands* on either side, each with a nipple. In young dogs these glands are not very prominent and look like little specks. In older females, particularly those who have had a litter of nursing puppies, the breasts may be more prominent and pendulous. In older, unspayed female dogs the mammary glands are prone to develop tumors, which are sometimes benign but are often highly malig-

nant. If an owner detects a lump in the area of the mammary glands, a veterinarian should be consulted immediately.

In addition to preventing accidental breeding and pregnancy, surgical neutering has many health and behavioral benefits for both male and female pet dogs. (See Chapter 2, "How to Keep a Dog's Body Healthy," page 13, and Chapter 3, "Normal Dog Behavior," page 29). Ideally, females are spayed (have an overiohysterectomy) before their first heat; males are generally castrated at about six to ten months of age. There is a discussion of early neutering in the following chapter.

Respiratory System

A dog's respiratory system is primarily responsible for bringing oxygen into his body to be carried into the bloodstream, and for eliminating carbon dioxide (the waste product of organ metabolism) from his body. The respiratory system starts with the *nose* or *mouth,* which delivers air to the *trachea,* or windpipe, a long hollow tube that begins at the back of the throat. Air is brought through the trachea to the *lungs* via *bronchi* and *bronchioles,* which come off the trachea like branches from a tree. The lungs are an elaborate network of membranes with very small blood vessels through which oxygen can pass and enter the bloodstream. Anything that interrupts this process of oxygenation, such as lung or bronchial disease, will cause difficulties because a dog's body will not get its required oxygen supply.

Urinary System

The urinary system of all mammals, including dogs, is primarily responsible for excreting waste products from the body and maintaining body water balance, assuring that the body has the proper amount of water at all times. The kidneys regulate this by removing water from urine before it is excreted, or by allowing more water to be passed in urine when it is excreted. Two very long thin tubes, called *ureters,* connect the kidneys to the *bladder.* The bladder is a hollow, muscular organ that stores urine and then contracts to excrete it outside the body through another tube called the *urethra.* Kidneys also provide important functions such as maintaining blood pressure, activating vitamin D for healthy bones, and stimulating the bone marrow to produce red blood cells.

Other Systems

Paws and claws: Dogs do not use their claws as weapons; they are mainly for foot protection, traction, and digging. If a dog does not wear down his claws on pavement they must be trimmed periodically (see "Grooming and Bathing," page 24).

A dog's footpads are thick and rough, but still must be protected from sharp objects such as broken glass, extremes in temperature, and from chemicals used in gardens and to melt ice and snow. Their sweat glands are located on the feet between their toes.

Anal glands: All dogs have anal glands, or sacs, on either side of the rectum, which secrete foul-smelling matter, usually when a dog defecates. Sometimes these glands become impacted and cause a dog to scoot on the ground on his rear end (see "Rectal Problems," pages 133 to 135, and "Straining to Move Bowels," pages 146 to 147). If this happens the glands must be man-

ually emptied by a veterinarian or experienced groomer. Anal glands may also become infected or abscessed and require medical attention.

How to Keep a Dog's Body Healthy

Just as is true in human health care, the best way to assure a dog's continuing health is by practicing commonsense care and preventive medicine. Regular checkups, immunizations against contagious diseases, nutrition that meets a dog's needs at each stage of her life, proper exercise, grooming, and generally good daily care combine to comprise a routine that will help a dog's body function at its maximum potential.

Choosing a Veterinarian

The first step to take in sensible preventive medicine is to choose a veterinarian who will care for a pet on a regular basis. It's a good idea to shop for a veterinarian *before* bringing home a new puppy or dog, because a thorough head-to-tail checkup is one of the very first procedures that should occur.

Although there are low-cost clinics that will perform most routine services such as yearly immunizations and boosters and simple neutering operations, most pet owners want a veterinarian with whom they can consult if some aspect of their pet's well-being troubles them. For this purpose a good general practitioner is the best choice. It is important for a veterinarian to get to know both pet and owner in order to be effective in assessing illnesses and disorders that may crop up later on in a dog's life.

Veterinarians vary greatly in ability and personality, just as human doctors do. For general pet care, probably the most important qualification for a veterinarian is an owner's ability to get along with and communicate well with the doctor. If something more complicated than regular care is needed, a general-practice veterinarian will usually refer a pet owner to a specialist in the area of concern, such as ophthalmology, cardiology, etc. It's a good idea to find out ahead of time if the veterinary practice being considered has access to these types of specialists, or to a large veterinary teaching facility or hospital with specialists on the staff.

The best sources of information about local veterinarians are pet-owning friends and neighbors. Breeders, groomers, and even pet-supply-store owners may also know of good local veterinarians. Many veterinarians are in group practice and share facilities and staff. Barring any of these resources, call the American Animal Hospital Association (AAHA) toll free (see page 211 for number). They have the names of member animal hospitals in all geographical areas. They set high standards for their animal hospital members in equipment, procedures, and physical facilities.

A great many animal hospitals are closed on Sundays, holidays, and during nighttime hours. For off-hour and holiday emergencies, several practices often join to establish a centrally located emergency clinic, manned by member veterinarians or employees of veterinarian hospitals on a rotating basis. If this arrangement is not satisfactory it may be best to find a veterinary practice in which one of the doctors is on call all of the time.

Once a preliminary decision is made to choose a particular veterinarian and/or practice, an appointment should be made for a checkup for a new puppy or dog as soon as possible after she comes home. If an owner finds the veterinarian is not satisfactory at that time, common sense dictates that another doctor be found. See below for more about what to expect on the first veterinary visit.

Choosing a Healthy Pet

A great deal of trouble and heartache can be avoided by choosing a puppy or dog that comes from healthy stock and is in good, robust health. In general, it's a good idea to ask to see the parents of the puppy, or at least the mother (bitch, dam). Her general health and condition are pretty good indicators of the puppy's health.

The first decision a potential dog owner has to make is what type of dog he wants and whether or not he wants a purebred or mixed-breed pet. The advantage of owning a purebred dog is predictability. An owner will know ahead of time what the dog's haircoat will be like, what size she will grow up to be, her grooming needs, exercise requirements, and general temperament tendencies.

A dog's temperament may be the most important factor for many potential owners. An older person may want a calm dog that's easy to walk and care for, for example, while a family with young children may opt for a gentle dog that won't bite if a child pulls her fur or steps on her foot. It is important, however, for potential owners to understand that there is a wide range of temperaments and personalities even within a given dog breed. There is no guarantee that an individual dog will act the same as another individual of the same breed. Veterinarians are familiar with the behavioral tendencies of particular dog breeds and can assist a potential owner with the selection of a pet.

The disadvantages of purebred ownership include the initial cost of a puppy, and the greater potential for a purebred dog to have inherited defects or disorders. To understand why inherited defects and disorders are more common among purebred than mixed-breed dogs, it is necessary to know a little something about genetics. Genetically inherited defects and diseases are usually transmitted from parent to offspring by genes that are abnormal. Because they are recessive they will not show up in offspring unless the offspring inherits two of these genes, one from each parent. It is possible for an animal to inherit only one recessive gene from one parent and not express the particular defect or disease. However, she will become a carrier of that defect or disease, and if bred to another animal that is also a carrier of the same defect or disease there is a 25 percent chance that a puppy will inherit recessive genes from both her parents and will develop that defect or disease. Therefore, the chances of a particular inheritable disease occurring in a particular dog increases in purebred dogs because the same recessive gene may be present in another member of that particular breed.

A mixed-breed dog has a much smaller chance of developing these types of inherited defects and diseases because of the decreased likelihood that two dogs of different breeds will carry the same recessive genes.

For first-time pet owners the most reliable source for a purebred dog can be a breeder or kennel. Breeders and kennels usually specialize in one or two breeds of dog and are extremely careful to preserve the quality of their animals. The American Kennel Club (AKC) will provide a list of registered breeders for most breeds of dogs (see page 211).

The best source for a mixed-breed dog is an animal shelter. Dogs end up in shelters for a variety of reasons and are often euthanized if not adopted. Saving a dog from death is often a good lesson for children and can increase the bond between animal and owner.

Whatever the source for a puppy, check to be sure she is in outwardly good health. Feel her entire body. A healthy puppy is solid-feeling. Her coat is shiny and her skin free from redness or irritation. Her eyes, ears, nose, and anal region are clean and free of caked matter or bad odors. The inside of her mouth is pink and her gums firm. Her footpads are firm and clean, and her nails are clean-looking and not torn or broken. She will not be coughing or sneezing, will have no mucoid nasal discharge, and will not have diarrhea. Healthy puppies are usually highly energetic when awake, very friendly, and not terribly shy.

As we mentioned above, the next step is to take her to the veterinarian as soon as possible to be sure she isn't harboring a disease or abnormal condition that is not outwardly noticeable.

A Veterinary Checkup

The first thing a veterinarian will do is look the puppy or dog over from head to tail, including the eyes and the insides of her ears and mouth. He'll feel her rib cage and abdomen for any swelling or abnormality, and check her skin, especially in the stomach and tail base area, for any signs of redness or possible flea bites. He will check the vulva of a female pup, or the prepuce, penis, and testicles of a male puppy. He'll weigh her and take her temperature. He'll also listen to her heart and lungs with a stethoscope.

Many young puppies have roundworms. Left unchecked, roundworms can cause a puppy to have diarrhea and eventually become very sick. They can also infect humans. Roundworm eggs are shed in the feces of an infected puppy, and will hatch to release infective larvae over time; if they are ingested by a human after hatching, they can migrate to various organs, most particularly the eye, where they will eventually cause blindness. Since most young children frequently put their unwashed hands into their mouths, this is especially important to be aware of if there are young children in the household. Because of the serious nature of roundworm infections in people it is essential that a puppy be routinely dewormed, even if no worms are visible in a stool sample. Dog feces should also be picked up and disposed of immediately because the eggs are not infectious until they hatch. Treatment with proper medication should be given several times at three-week intervals, usually at the same time immunizations are given. The medication is safe, effective, and not expensive.

If a dog or puppy seems to be in general good health, the next step is to establish an immunization schedule. Puppies need to be vaccinated against infectious diseases every few weeks to be fully protected (see Chart 1, opposite). Be sure to ask the veterinarian at what stage in the immunization process it will be safe to allow a puppy outdoors, where they may contact other dogs or dog viruses.

Immunity to a disease is not a lifetime condition but must be reinforced regularly for a dog to be protected. Adult dogs need revaccination, so-called booster shots, in order to retain immunity from disease. In many cases this is an annual requirement and should coincide with a yearly head-to-toe checkup. See page 18 for an adult dog's booster schedule. Even if a dog never leaves her own home she should be protected from dangerous infectious diseases. She can be exposed to disease from infectious feces brought in on people's shoes, by airborne viruses, by bacteria carried on clothing and hands, by insect carriers, and by chance encounters with other dogs and their waste on visits to the veterinarian or stays in a kennel.

How Do Vaccinations Work, and What Do They Prevent?

Vaccinations help a dog's body develop *antibodies,* which fight off specific infectious diseases by awakening the body's immune system to the particular bacteria or virus that causes the disease when it invades the animal's body. An antibody is manufactured in the dog's body when it is exposed to the disease organism in the vaccine. Vaccines are used to prevent diseases, not treat them, and will do no good if a dog is already infected with a disease.

Protection against canine distemper, hepatitis, and parainfluenza is combined in one vaccine (DHP); canine parvovirus may be a separate vaccine or combined with DHP. Rabies is a separate vaccine. Heartworm disease is prevented by oral medication (see below). More about all of these diseases in Chapter 5, "Contagious and Infectious Diseases."

One thing for owners to remember is that various diseases have different *incubation periods,* or lapses in time between exposure to the disease and the actual outbreak. During the incubation period of a disease the animal will show no signs of illness. It isn't until the disease has spread throughout a dog's body that she will become visibly ill. This is especially true in young puppies, particularly if they have not been given good health care previously. Sometimes seemingly healthy puppies that are in the process of being immunized can sicken and even die

Chart 1:
RECOMMENDED VACCINATIONS FOR ALL PUPPIES

(Note: The vaccines contained in "puppy shots" may vary according to individual veterinarians. These are the vaccinations we believe all puppies should have.)

Disease	6–8 wks.*	9–12 wks.	13–15 wks.	16+ wks.
Parvovirus	+	+	+	+
Distemper/Hepatitis Parainfluenza (DHP)	+	+	+	
Rabies			+	

*Not every veterinarian begins vaccinations this early.

DHP and Parvovirus immunizations for puppies should be given every 2–4 weeks from the time they are started until the pup reaches the appropriate age.

Chart 2:
OTHER VACCINATIONS THAT ARE AVAILABLE FOR PUPPIES

These vaccinations are not routinely given in all areas. A veterinarian will recommend them in those geographic areas where the incidence of the disease warrants immunization.

Disease	6–8 wks.	9–12 wks.	13–15 wks.
Coronavirus*	+	+	+
Leptospirosis*	+	+	+
Lyme disease	+	+	+
Nasal bordetella*	+	+	+

*Required by some boarding kennels.

because they were infected with a disease before vaccines were started. It is important to start puppy immunizations soon after weaning. Puppies are given some antibodies by their mothers that protect them for a short, undetermined time. Vaccines will not be effective when a puppy is still protected by maternal antibodies, but it is impossible to know when the maternal antibodies will disappear. This is why a series of vaccinations are used for puppies, to ensure that a vaccine is given when a puppy needs it.

There is currently a controversy about canine immunizations. Nobody knows for sure how long immunity lasts in adult dogs. A growing number of people believe dogs are being vaccinated too frequently and do not need yearly boosters. Opponents are afraid that if the frequency of vaccinations is reduced, the result will be the return of many serious canine diseases. At the time of this writing, we believe that animal vaccination for most diseases is the safest approach and still recom-

Chart 3:
RECOMMENDED VACCINATIONS FOR ALL ADULT DOGS

(Note: DHP and Parvovirus vaccines should be given one year after the last puppy immunizations. The first rabies vaccination is good for only one year, no matter what type of vaccine is used.)

Disease	Yearly	Every 1–3 years depending on type of vaccine used and local laws
Distemper/Hepatitis/ Parainfluenza (DHP)	+	
Parvovirus	+	
Rabies		+

Chart 4:
OPTIONAL VACCINATIONS FOR ADULT DOGS

The following vaccinations are available for dogs and should be given in areas where the incidence of the disease is high, according to the veterinarian's discretion.

Coronavirus*

Leptospirosis

Lyme disease

Nasal bordetella*

*Required by some boarding kennels.

mend following the schedules found on pages 17 and 18.

Dogs are protected against *heartworm disease* with oral medication rather than by vaccination. Heartworm disease, transmitted by mosquitoes from an infected dog to a healthy dog, also goes through an incubation period. Therefore, a blood test is taken, yearly in most parts of the country, to be sure there is no heartworm present in a dog's body before she is given preventative heartworm medication. Young puppies are an exception. They do not need the test because they have not had time to develop heartworms. Puppies should be started on the oral preventative, as prescribed by the veterinarian.

Spaying and Neutering

At the same time the veterinarian sets up an immunization schedule he will probably want to discuss the benefits of spaying or neutering a pet dog.

If an owner does not want to breed a pet dog, an overiohysterectomy (OHE, "spay") of a female dog or castration ("neutering," "altering") of a male dog are desirable for a number of reasons, both behavioral and physical. In both cases, of course, these operations prevent the accidental conception and birth of unwanted litters of puppies.

For a female dog, an OHE also prevents the occurrence of heat periods, which are often accompanied by a bloody vaginal discharge, restless behavior, irritability, and the inevitable gathering of eager would-be male suitors. Depending on the breed of dog, the operation is ideally performed at six to seven months, before a female's first heat period, when she is almost full-grown. When the operation is done at this age it dramati-

cally lessens the risk of her developing mammary gland (breast) cancer, one of the most common malignancies in dogs. The longer the OHE is delayed, the higher the risk that mammary gland cancer will develop later in the dog's life. An older dog who has not had an OHE may also develop a serious, life-threatening uterine infection (pyometra), which will need to be treated surgically (see pages 51 and 113).

Although an OHE is a major abdominal operation, modern medical techniques have made it painless and relatively uncomplicated when performed by a competent veterinarian. A dog will usually stay in the hospital overnight after an OHE to be certain she has come out of the anesthetic well and is comfortable. After a day or two of quiet rest at home, she usually shows no signs of discomfort. Complications rarely occur, but if a dog should show signs of discomfort or the incision becomes red or irritated, the veterinarian should be consulted.

For a male dog, a neutering operation cuts down dramatically on roaming behavior, and can reduce aggressive behavior (see Chapter 3, pages 36 to 37 and page 40). The operation is usually performed at around six to ten months of age, when the dog is sexually mature. It can be done when a dog is older, but by this time bad habits such as roaming and aggressiveness are more ingrained and difficult to change. Just as testosterone, the male sex hormone, can affect aggressive behavior, it can also affect health. Some testosterone-related health problems are benign prostate hypertropy—prostatitis, perineal hernias (page 134), perianal gland tumors (page 134), and hair loss (see "Skin Disorders," pages 140 to 145). Testicular cancer can also occur, especially in older intact (noncastrated) dogs; the treatment of choice is castration (see pages 123 and 134).

The neutering operation is less invasive than an OHE and the dog is sometimes allowed to go home the same day. Complications are rare. The most common problem is swelling of the scrotum due to irritation or bleeding. If this occurs, the veterinarian will be able to advise what steps to take.

In recent years many animal shelters have begun to neuter young puppies before they are adopted in order to avoid the birth of more unwanted puppies. So far, early neutering has proved to be safe and effective. However, not enough time has elapsed since this procedure was begun to find out if there are any negative long-term health effects. If a puppy from a shelter has already been castrated or had an OHE, there is probably nothing for a prospective owner to worry about. If the procedure has not already been done, it is best to perform the surgeries at the recommended ages.

What About Weight Gain After Spaying or Neutering?

Many owners continue to believe the myth that spaying or neutering a dog inevitably leads to weight gain. Rather, because the operations are usually performed just as a dog is maturing—going from puberty to adulthood—she or he is full-grown and often less active and requires fewer extra calories for growth.

The primary culprits in weight gain after spaying or neutering are too many calories for that stage in a dog's life and not enough exercise. If an owner continues to feed a young dog the same amount of food she was receiving when she was six months old, she will inevitably gain weight. The same holds true for exercise, which we'll discuss later in this chapter. Young puppies are pretty much self-starters as far as exercise is

concerned. As they become older, many dogs require more encouragement from their owners in order to get enough exercise to burn off excess calories. See "Exercise," page 22.

Providing Good Nutrition

Almost all dogs enjoy eating and will eat just about any food they can get hold of. Feeding a pet dog and watching her enjoy her food can be a great pleasure for an owner. However, in order for a dog to grow well, with strong bones, muscles, and teeth, and in order to maintain her good health and energy, a dog's nutritional needs must be met by feeding her a complete, balanced diet designed for dogs. Dogs require a proper balance of carbohydrates, fats, and protein, along with vitamins and minerals, just as all mammals do. In general, "people food" does not meet a dog's nutritional requirements. People have different requirements than dogs do, and a different ability to utilize and absorb nutrients.

There are complete and balanced diets designed specifically for dogs at all stages of their lives and under all conditions, including illness. During the past twenty years knowledge of dogs' nutritional needs has grown a great deal, and there are many excellent dog foods available, in grocery stores, specialty pet stores, veterinarian offices, and even grooming establishments.

To avoid upsets a new puppy or dog should be fed whatever type of food she has been used to eating. Breeders often send home a "care package" with several days' supply of food to start a puppy off right. If it becomes necessary, or desirable, to change diets, it's best to do so gradually, by mixing a small amount of new food with whatever a dog is accustomed to. If she accepts the mix well, without any intestinal upset, increase the new food gradually each day until the dog is eating the new diet exclusively. Most dogs do well eating the same food every day, as long as it's complete and balanced. It isn't necessary or even desirable to vary a dog's diet—the result is often a bout of diarrhea or vomiting. The same holds true of adding treats from the table. Treats designed for dogs, such as biscuits, are all right as long as too many aren't given, which will cause a dog to gain excessive weight. A good rule of thumb is that snacks or treats should not exceed 10 to15 percent of a dog's daily diet.

Kinds of Dog Food

There are several basic kinds of dog food: dry, semimoist, and canned. There are special diets for special needs, such as puppy food, food for dogs under severe stress, old dogs, fat dogs, and dogs with certain medical conditions. There are also dog treats, crunchy biscuit types and chewy treats. Some foods are often fed in conjunction with each other, such as canned and dry.

Avoiding Excessive Weight Gain

It is difficult to say exactly how much to feed an individual dog in order to prevent excessive weight gain; a lot depends on the dog's basic metabolism, age, and the amount of exercise she gets. Manufacturers' recommendations for quantities of food per day, given on pet food labels, usually exceed the amounts recommended by veterinarians. It is interesting to note that small dogs require more calories per pound of body weight than do large breeds.

There are inexpensive dry maintenance diets that are often used by kennels. Sometimes owners prefer them over richer foods because they can safely be left out all day for free-choice feeding; due to their lack of taste appeal, a dog will not overeat. Other dry dog foods, canned foods, and puppy foods that are high in calories and nutrition contain flavor enhancers. They are too appealing to be left out for free-choice feeding, because they will cause a dog to overeat and gain too much weight.

The veterinarian will weigh a dog each time she comes into the office and will be able to advise an owner if the dog is gaining too much weight. A good at-home test to see if a dog is overweight is by feeling her ribs. With both thumbs resting on her backbone, feel her ribs on either side of her body. If she is too fat, her ribs can barely be felt under a layer of fat. If she's too thin, the sharp edge of each rib can be felt.

Feeding a Puppy

There are foods available on the market that are designed to meet a puppy's special nutritional needs. Until they are about six months of age, puppies require twice as many calories per pound than do adult dogs of the same breed. This amount can usually be reduced to about one and a half times as much as an adult's intake at six months; then to just slightly over an adult dog's ration when the pup has reached approximately 80 percent of her full growth. Puppies also require specific nutrients to grow properly and develop strong bones, teeth, muscles, and organs. Owners should know, however, that adult dog foods labeled "complete and balanced for all life stages" are nutritious enough for puppies, or that could not appear on the label.

In order to obtain needed calories it is usually recommended that owners divide puppies' rations into three or four meals a day until they are at least half grown. After that the number of feedings can be reduced gradually until the dog is about a year old, at which time one meal a day is the usual recommendation. Sometimes small breeds do better with two small meals a day. The veterinarian will usually set up a feeding schedule based on the pup's breed, size, and rate of growth or weight gain. See Table 1, right, for the results of deficiencies in a puppy's diet. Overfeeding of puppies can cause serious skeletal problems by increasing their growth rate.

Supplements

There are a number of vitamin and mineral supplements on the market. Most of these are in tablet form and are very appealing to dogs. Some owners give bonemeal and/or calcium supplements to growing puppies. If a puppy or dog is eating a complete and balanced diet designed for dogs, supplements should not be given, except under a doctor's orders. Oversupplementation can upset a dog's nutritional balance; in large-breed growing puppies, it can cause serious skeletal problems.

Water

Fresh water should be available to dogs all of the time. As long as water is available, dogs in good health will drink the proper amount to flush waste from their bodies, carry nutrients throughout their bodies, and keep their body fluids at the proper level. There are some medical conditions that lead to overdrinking (see page 148).

Foods to Avoid

There are some "people foods" that can make a dog sick and should be avoided. One of many people's favorites, chocolate, is also very attractive to dogs. It can make a dog very sick and, depending on her size and the amount of chocolate she eats, can even kill her. Chocolate contains a substance called theobromine, which can cause a form of intoxication in dogs, including vomiting, incontinence, and agitation, that in severe cases may escalate to seizures and death. The majority of calls received by veterinarians about chocolate poisoning in dogs occur around holiday times, when owners tend to want to share their goodies with their pets. If a dog is known to have eaten chocolate and becomes ill, seek veterinary help right away (see "Poisoning," pages 47 to 48).

Another popular human food that is not good for dogs is onions. While a dog is not likely to consume a plain onion, she may go for a bit of leftover meat smothered in onions. Too many onions, raw or cooked, can damage a dog's red blood cells and cause them to burst. Eventually, the dog will become anemic; she may also vomit or act weak. Again, veterinary help should be sought right away if a dog is known to have eaten onions. Prompt action can save the dog's life (see page 137).

A class of foods to avoid for an adult dog are dairy products. Milk and cheese are often poorly digested by many adult dogs and may give them diarrhea. (The exception is cottage cheese, which is digestible and may be prescribed for certain conditions.) No medical treatment is usually necessary once the dog no longer eats dairy products, unless the diarrhea persists (see "Diarrhea," pages 50 and 101 to 105).

Exercise

Just as it is difficult to recommend an exact amount of food to give a dog, it is hard to say exactly how much exercise a specific dog requires. One good measure to determine whether or not a dog is getting sufficient exercise

Table 1: CONDITIONS RESULTING FROM SOME DEFICIENCIES IN A PUPPY'S DIET	
Nutrient	**Resulting Condition if Deficient**
Calories (energy)	Thin body; poor haircoat; slow growth; lack of growth; susceptibility to bacterial infection and parasitic invasion.
Fat and essential fatty acids	Coarse, dry coat; skin lesions; infection.
Protein and amino acids	Severe lack of growth; weight loss; muscle wasting; coarse, dry coat.
Minerals	
Calcium and phosphorus	Convulsions; poor growth; soft bones; fractures.
Potassium	Poor growth; restlessness; muscular paralysis; dehydration; damage to internal organs.
Sodium and chloride	Retarded growth; exhaustion; decreased water intake; dry skin; hair loss.
Magnesium	Loss of appetite; poor weight gain; lack of coordination; irritability; convulsions.
Iron	Anemia.
Zinc	Retarded weight gain; skin lesions.
Iodine	Goiter; skin and skeletal deformities; timidity; drowsiness.
Vitamins	
Fat-soluble	Rarely deficient; excess can be toxic.
A	Bone and nerve impairment; eye and skin problems; weight loss.
D (must be in balance with calcium and phosphorus)	Soft bones; fractures.
E	Muscle weakness; impaired immune response; retinal degeneration.
Water-soluble	
B-complex	Loss of appetite; failure to grow; weight loss; weakness; anemia; susceptibility to infection.

Based on: *Nutrient Requirements of Dogs,* revised 1985. © 1985 by the National Academy of Sciences.

is to assess her weight. See "Avoiding Excessive Weight Gain," page 21.

A growing puppy needs no supplementary exercise, and owners should be careful not to allow a puppy to jump excessively. Large, heavy breeds especially are susceptible to joint and bone injuries if they are allowed to play too roughly or wildly. As a dog becomes a senior citizen she will require less vigorous exercise, and care should be taken not to tire her out or aggravate arthritis, if present. Although regular daily exercise can help an obese dog lose weight, overweight dogs of all ages must be exercised in gradual increments in order not to damage their cardiovascular systems and joints.

Generally, healthy adult dogs need daily exercise, not only to avoid weight gain but for entertainment and stimulation and to get rid of excess energy. Sufficient exercise can help break most dogs of destructive behavior in the house. Many dogs, especially small ones, seem to be constantly on the move. They run around the house a lot and get quite a bit of exercise that way. Dogs that live with energetic children also get a lot of exercise by just romping with their families. Some dog breeds were developed over the years to work hard. Terriers, hunting, and retrieving dogs fall into this category. They usually have a great deal of energy and stamina and need to be exercised more than quieter types that have been bred solely as companion pets.

In general, dogs with short legs, such as dachshunds and very small toys, can get enough exercise just running around the yard, or on a short walk. Longer-legged breeds need a lot more rigorous, daily exercise in order to stay in shape.

Exercise Guidelines

- If a dog is going to be asked to indulge in strenuous exercise, she should be conditioned gradually, just as a human athlete would be. Be sure to have a dog checked by the veterinarian before a vigorous exercise program begins.
- Because dogs want to please, they will often continue to exercise when at the point of exhaustion, especially in hot weather. An owner should be aware of this and check a dog for excessive panting, apparent fatigue, loss of color in gums, and/or a vacant stare.
- Never exercise a dog strenuously less than two hours after she eats a big meal.

Grooming and Bathing

An important routine to establish with a dog is regular coat care. Depending on the type of haircoat a dog has, a daily or twice-weekly grooming session will keep her coat clean and free from snarls and mats, remove loose hair that will otherwise end up on the carpet or furniture, and help promote healthy skin. Puppies should become used to being combed and brushed as early as possible in their lives. Most dogs enjoy the process and it also gives an owner a good chance to look a dog over for any signs of problems such as parasites, lumps, bumps, rashes, or even small wounds underneath the fur that may not be immediately visible. During grooming it's a good idea to occasionally look a dog completely over: check the insides of her ears, her feet and footpads, and the inside of her mouth.

Some dogs enjoy every aspect of grooming, except when it comes to feet and legs. Usually it's the restraint of her feet that a dog objects to. Grooming may work better if, instead of grasping the paws, an owner allows a dog to rest her paws one at a time in the owner's hand and then gently brushes them. The other areas of a dog's body that are often very sensitive are her face, tummy, ears, and tail area. These sensitive spots should be stroked softly and then brushed or combed very gently. If these tender areas are hurt during grooming, a dog's confidence in her owner may be destroyed. If a dog cries out when her ears are touched, or refuses even gentle brushing, an owner should suspect an ear infection (see pages 106 to 108).

Some kinds of haircoat require special handling. If a longhaired dog develops mats or tangles in her coat, they should be gently worked out by hand, or clipped out, never pulled or yanked. Double-coated dogs such as collies and German shepherds should be brushed against the grain from the skin outward, to remove loose hairs. Dogs with curly hair, like poodles, have to be periodically trimmed, and some wirehaireds such as schnauzers and many terriers usually have their coats plucked to remove excess hair approximately twice a year. Many owners opt to perform these grooming processes themselves. In order to learn how to do this properly it is usually necessary to take a class or work with a professional groomer. Picture books about grooming really don't do a good enough instructional job, although there are useful videos that demonstrate the specific grooming processes for particular breeds of dogs. The majority of pet owners prefer to go to professional groomers, who will not only groom a dog but bathe her, clip her nails, and generally make the dog look and feel good.

If a dog doesn't wear her nails down on pavement, they must be clipped on a regular basis. Nails that are allowed to grow too long may become ingrown, can cause foot problems,

and may catch on things or break. Groomers and veterinarians usually perform this service whenever a dog visits. If an owner decides to clip a dog's nails himself, it's best to learn how to do it correctly from a professional.

Bathing a Dog

Breeders and veterinarians can advise new dog owners as to the bathing needs of most dogs. Many dogs never need a bath, but those with long hair should be bathed at least every six to eight weeks. Dogs with smooth, oily coats, such as Labrador retrievers, usually don't require frequent bathing—regular brushing will keep their coats clean. Those with very heavy coats, or double coats, need to be bathed only a couple of times a year; also it can be difficult to dry them thoroughly. Of course, circumstances can make it essential for a dog to have a bath, such as an encounter with a skunk, or a roll in something especially foul-smelling. Dogs who sleep in owners' bedrooms or on their beds may require fairly frequent baths in order to be good-smelling companions.

Owners need to be careful not to chill a dog. Baths should be given in warm, draft-free areas. In warm weather a dog can be bathed outdoors, but it may be difficult to arrange for warm water outside. A quality shampoo made especially for dogs usually works well, but if a dog has particularly sensitive skin, a human or baby shampoo may be better. It is essential to rinse all of the shampoo out of a dog's coat, or her skin will become irritated and itch. A small amount of mild dog-coat conditioner will help make it easier to comb out a longhaired dog. After the bath allow the dog to shake to rid herself of excess moisture and then rub her vigorously with terry towels. Comb and brush the dog, and be sure she stays in a warm, draft-free area until she is completely dry (check the skin underneath the thickest part of her coat).

Owners often find it easier to have a dog professionally bathed on a regular basis. If a dog is particularly difficult to handle, or particularly large, this may be the only practical option.

Fleas and Ticks

If a dog is hosting either fleas or ticks, they will be visible during grooming and/or bathing.

These parasites are not difficult to recognize. Fleas like the thick fur around a dog's neck and at the base of the spine where it meets the tail. They also can sometimes be seen in the groin area or armpits. Sometimes the fleas themselves can be seen—tiny dark brown insects that jump very high and fast or scurry through the coat. Usually what an owner will see is flea exudate (waste, or "flea dirt") in the form of tiny black specks. If a flea infestation is allowed to go unchecked it can lead not only to serious skin problems but may cause a dog to become anemic. The anemia can be severe and life-threatening in young puppies. Fleas act as hosts to tapeworm larvae, so if a dog ingests infected fleas it can lead to a tapeworm infestation (see page 103).

When they are not engorged with blood ticks are tiny, flat, dark brown bugs with legs. When they are full of blood they swell up and look like tan- or gray-colored beans. Initially,

they may be loose in a dog's fur, but they then adhere to a dog, suck her blood, and become engorged. They attach themselves very firmly and must be removed by pinching them off close to the skin. Ticks are carriers of several diseases that can be dangerous and even fatal to dogs, including Rocky Mountain spotted fever, ehrlichiosis, and Lyme disease (see pages 61 and 62). Since some of these diseases are also contagious to people, gloves should be worn when ticks are removed. It is also important to note that deer ticks, which carry Lyme disease, are much smaller than the normal brown dog tick. They can be very difficult to detect on dogs.

There are now excellent products on the market that either repel these parasites or break down their reproductive cycle by preventing them from laying viable eggs. The veterinarian will give advice on the best method to use in a given area. When parasites are already present, a flea and tick bath, or "dip," is generally effective in removing existing pests from a dog. If a dog should become infested, however, it is important to remember that these parasites do not live on dogs, but simply *feed* on them. If the only step taken is to kill the parasites already on the dog, more will simply return, because they live in the environment, in the house and yard. In order to control a flea or tick population, the eggs and larvae must be killed, as well as the adult parasites. There are a number of different ways to accomplish this. A veterinarian will be able to help determine the best way to eliminate these pests in a given climatic and geographic area.

Tooth Care

Veterinarians recommend regular tooth care for all dogs, but especially for smaller breeds, which often develop tooth and gum

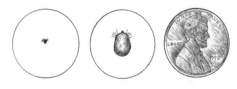

Left: An unengorged tick. Center: An engorged tick.

problems when they grow older. Without proper care a dog's teeth will develop tartar, which inevitably will lead to gum disease and tooth loss.

Nowadays there are toothbrushes and toothpaste made expressly for dogs that are available from veterinarians and pet specialty stores. Human toothpaste is not good for dogs. They don't like it because it foams too much, and has the wrong flavor for dogs. If dog toothpaste isn't available, a slightly moistened mix of baking soda and salt will do just as well. Also, a small child's toothbrush with soft-to-medium bristles works the same as one made for dogs.

Just as with other grooming routines, the earlier a puppy becomes used to having her teeth cleaned, the easier it will be. Some dog dentifrice kits contain a finger brush to start with—a flexible rubber tube with a rough tip that slips over the index finger. If this is not available use a rough terry cloth wrapped around a finger and gently rub the dog's teeth, starting at the gum and working toward the tooth tip. Once a puppy is used to having her teeth cleaned this way, a brush can be introduced. This routine should be performed approximately once a week; the veterinarian will recommend more frequent brushings if needed.

If a grown dog has not been having her teeth cleaned regularly, the veterinarian should look at her teeth and scale them to remove built-up tartar before a brushing routine at home is begun. Hand scaling on a dog that is awake is insufficient. A thorough dental prophylaxis involves general anesthesia and ultrasonographic scaling followed by polishing.

If there is any redness or bleeding of the gums or anything else that doesn't look right, a veterinarian should see the dog's mouth right away. The same, of course, holds true in the case of broken, loose, or sensitive teeth and a foul mouth odor.

Other Important Care Procedures

Owners need to remember that dogs, like all other animals, need to know what to expect. They are happiest when they know when they are going to be fed, taken out, played with, and put to bed. A rigid routine isn't necessary, but dogs thrive best when care routines occur on a more or less regular basis.

Of course, unexpected things happen in any household that may change a routine, delay a feeding or a walk, for instance. Once a dog is an adult she is usually able to handle occasional lapses in everyday schedules as long as they don't happen all the time. Owners who anticipate regular late working hours or other circumstances that will leave a dog alone for too long should arrange for a sitter, or walker, to come to the house and take care of the dog's needs. More about this in Chapter 3, "Normal Dog Behavior."

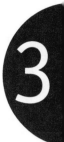

Normal Dog

Behavior

Most dogs are affectionate companions by nature
and give completely nonjudgmental loyalty to
their owners. The fact that, over the years, dogs
have learned to perform a number of difficult and
complex tasks that help their owners and others
is testament to their innate ability to learn and
desire to please their masters.

In this chapter we will describe normal dog
behavior so a first-time owner will know what to
expect. We will also cover several inappropriate
canine behaviors that frequently trouble owners
and provide some suggestions about how to deal
with them.

Social Behavior of Dogs

Probably the single most important
thing for dog owners to understand is that
domestic dogs' ancestors—wolves—live in packs
and, despite domestication, dogs have retained

their pack instincts. To them, humans are part of their pack.

Another thing for owners to consider is that all puppies go through periods of socialization at various times during their growing up. One of the most critical periods, when a puppy learns to socialize with his littermates, is between the age of four and fourteen weeks. Pups that are denied socialization with other dogs for whatever reason are apt to become either overly timid or aggressive with other dogs when they grow up. Positive socialization with humans is also critical for puppies during the same early weeks of life if they are going to become good pets.

A grown dog that has not had good experiences with a variety of humans as a puppy will be difficult to train because he will either be timid or dominating. If he is overly timid, he will react to even the mildest correction with cringing, submissive behavior. If he is overly dominating he will respond to correction and/or discipline with aggressive behavior. Responsible breeders never allow a pup to be taken home before at least eight weeks of age so that he has been well socialized both to other dogs and to humans during this critical period.

If a puppy has been well socialized to other dogs and to people he will generally be good-tempered and anxious to please. A lot of a dog's behavior depends on breed characteristics and on the dog's individual genetics, of course. People have selectively bred dogs for particular purposes such as hunting, herding, or guarding. We should not be surprised when the hunter hunts the cat, the herder herds the guests out the door, or the guard dog guards the front door from the meter reader, the mail carrier, and even one's own father.

Sleeping Behavior

Pet dogs that are kept indoors usually sleep through the night. This may be in response to the sleep patterns of their owners. Dogs kept tied up outdoors and/or free-roaming dogs tend to be most active at dawn and just before sunset.

Dogs left alone at home during the day, whether crated or not, usually spend at least half of the day sleeping, interspersed with short (half-hour to two-hour) activity periods. Their sleep alternates between light, or wakeful, sleep (slow wave sleep, or SWS) and deep (REM) sleep. In humans, REM sleep is dream sleep and it appears to be the same for dogs. Owners often notice a sleeping dog whimpering softly or moving his legs slightly as if he's dreaming.

Puppies generally maintain contact with littermates when sleeping. A newly adopted pup may feel less lonely the first few nights he sleeps alone in his new home if he is given a warm hot water bottle or old towel or sweater for "contact."

Eating Behavior

Dogs tend to gulp their food without chewing it thoroughly. They usually eat very quickly—some owners joke that they "inhale" their meals.

Gulping behavior can lead to problems when walking a dog in areas where there is garbage on the street, or in the country, where there may be carrion. A dog will grab and quickly swallow anything he can find to eat before an owner can stop him, even if it is sometimes spoiled or dangerous. This habit can make a dog extremely sick. One of the first things an owner should teach a pet is either the "Leave It!" command, in which a dog is conditioned not to pick up anything in his mouth, or the "Drop It!" command, in which a dog is taught to let go of, or allow his owner to take away, any object or food he may have in his mouth. These commands are often taught in obedience classes, but an owner can quite easily teach them to a pet using praise and reward when the dog obeys. See also "Communicating with a Dog," page 35.

Except for some tiny toy breeds and coursing breeds, most dogs enjoy eating and will often seem to be hungry all the time. An owner may interpret this as a sign she isn't feeding her dog enough. If she increases a dog's rations too much or feeds him table scraps or treats every time the dog begs for food, it may lead quickly to obesity, which is a serious health threat. A dog should be fed only the amount of food that keeps him in good condition. A veterinarian or breeder can recommend the proper diet, suitable for the dog's breed, activity level, and the environment in which he lives. For more about this, see Chapter 2, page 21, "Avoiding Excessive Weight Gain."

Territorial Behavior

Dogs tend to be territorial by nature, just as wolves are. A dog's idea of "his" territory may not coincide with what we consider our property lines. As a dog becomes mature he may expand his territory to include first the sidewalk in front of his lawn, and then gradually the entire block or street. The syndrome of expanding territory to a wider and wider area is especially prevalent in intact, unneutered males.

Individual dogs will defend their territories with different degrees of fervor. Some dogs simply bark when their territory is invaded, but others will bite, especially if their warning bark is ignored and a person or another dog continues to

come farther into the territory. This is especially true in breeds that have been bred selectively to be aggressive guard dogs, such as chows, Akitas, shepherds, rottweilers, and pit bulls, to name a few.

Dogs often "mark" their territories with urine. Males mark more commonly than females, but spayed females may also mark. Although behaviorists don't know for sure exactly what dogs are communicating to each other, dogs do seem to be able to gain information from other dogs' markings. They can differentiate between those of males and females, females in estrus or not, and even between those of individual dogs.

Dogs also frequently scratch the ground after urinating or defecating. This is apparently not a scent marking because there is very little scent in dogs' feet. No one really knows why they do this, but it's thought by some that this is a visual sign that is more noticeable from a distance than the smell of urine or feces, enabling another dog to perceive the marking from farther away. It may also spread the odor of the urine or feces.

Canine Communications

Canines communicate within pack society by using body language that is readily understood by all individual pack members. Dogs try to communicate with their owners in the same way. But when their body language is misunderstood or ignored by humans they will escalate their actions just the way an English-speaking person in a foreign country will often speak louder and louder when his words aren't understood.

For example, a dog that's feeling aggressive will stand in a rigid posture with tail extended

Table 2:
CANINE BODY LANGUAGE

	Body	Tail	Ears	Eyes	Vocalization
Chase preparation	Tense, crouched, knees and elbows bent	Extended straight behind the body	Perked up, pointing forward	Wide open, looking at moving object or person	Perhaps a soft, excited whine
Dominance aggression	Rigid; hair up on neck and back	Rigid; extended up over back; sometimes wagging in small motions	Pricked	Wide open, staring; sometimes narrowed	Loud barking; snarling; growling
Fear	Tense, crouched low; trembling; possible emptying of anal sacs	Low, between rear legs	Flattened against head	Pupils dilated; avoids direct eye contact	Low, threatening growl
Playfulness	Front of body lowered, rear up, or sitting with paw extended and head cocked to the side; pawing side of face; sometimes bouncing and running excitedly in circles	Wagging hard	Perked up	Wide open, cheerful-looking	Excited barking, whining, play growling
Submission	Low; lying on back, belly showing; possible urination	Low, between rear legs	Flattened against head	Averted	None, or low, worried whining/ whimpering

upward stiffly. If a person doesn't understand this is an aggressive posture and continues to approach, the dog makes his message clearer by raising the hairs on the back of his neck, growl-ing, or showing his teeth. Ultimately, if his mes-sage is still not heeded, the dog may attack and bite.

The tail of a frightened dog will be between his legs and his ears will be flattened. He'll crouch low to the ground and avert his eyes. With this posture he's saying, "I'm afraid. Please leave me alone, you're scaring me." If his message is ignored and a human or another dog continues

A dog standing in a normal, relaxed posture

A dog using body language to clearly demonstrate dominance aggression

to approach, the dog may take the next step and bite to protect himself.

In both of these instances, when a miscommunication occurs, the dog is reacting normally, but the results may be serious. It is important for dog owners to learn to recognize canine body language in order to interact successfully with their pets.

OTHER TYPICAL CANINE BODY LANGUAGE

Just as a submissive wolf will signal to a dominant pack member, a submissive dog that wants to let his owner know she's the boss will lie flat on the ground, or on his back, belly up, ears flattened, and eyes averted. When the owner comes closer the dog often urinates a small amount to emphasize his submission. If an owner then becomes angry at this action, the dog is completely confused. If he could talk he would say, "I am showing you I'm completely abject and submissive to you. Why do you keep on threatening me?"

A dog that wants to play will signal his joyful intent by lowering his front legs, rear end sticking up in the air. This is known as a "play bow." The dog may then bounce up and down or

This dog has assumed a fearfully submissive attitude

A typical "play bow"

circle around excitedly. He may make short barks or whine and growl. His ears will be up and his tail wagging at the same time. Some dogs also paw at their noses—another play signal.

Owners must be careful not to confuse a play bow with a similar posture that a dog may take when his abdomen is sore (see page 40). That posture is often referred to as "praying," that is, praying that the pain will go away. The difference is usually obvious because a dog in pain will not look merry or wag his tail.

A dog will also give a clear indication when he's about to chase someone or something. His ears will be perked forward and his body will be tense. He'll be crouched, knees and elbows flexed, ready to begin running. This is predatory posture.

These are a few of the more common postures dogs use to communicate with their owners. An observant owner will soon learn to interpret her own dog's body language.

VOCALIZATION

Dogs communicate vocally by barking, howling, whining, and growling.

Wolves do not bark often, but they do howl as a pack activity and perhaps to locate one another. Dog breeds that are closely related to wolves, such as malamutes and huskies, also howl frequently, as do some hounds. Pet dogs often get into the habit of barking to warn others off their territory. Terriers are especially apt to bark at anyone who walks by, especially other dogs or animals. Because of dogs' acute hearing and sense of smell, owners are often not aware another animal is anywhere near.

Puppies whine to get their mothers' attention. Grown pet dogs usually whine if they are lonely and want their owners' attention, or when they are prevented from joining in family activity by a gate or closed door. They may also whine if they don't feel well or are in pain, again communicating a need for attention.

Growling is usually an aggressive warning vocalization in dogs. But dogs will also emit what is called a "play growl," accompanied by playful body language (see page 32).

Communicating with a Dog

Once an owner fully realizes that her dog really doesn't understand spoken language, it becomes clear a dog needs to be *shown* what's wanted rather than *told*. A dog doesn't know what's wanted until he is clearly shown. Almost all dogs want to please their owners and will look intently at them for clues as to how to behave.

For example, if an owner wants her dog to learn to sit on command, she should wait until she sees the dog is about to sit, say "Sit," and then praise the dog for sitting. Soon the dog will learn to associate the word *sit* with the action.

This commonsense approach can be applied to many training situations as long as an owner continuously bears in mind that the dog cannot understand what's being said to him, but must be shown again and again and praised whenever he gets it right.

Tone of voice also plays an important role in helping a dog understand what's wanted. "Good dog," said in an upbeat, cheerful tone of voice, immediately conveys the desired message. But "no" or "bad dog" said in the same tone will also communicate approval. Owners should remember that the manner in which words are said means something to a dog, not the actual words used.

Elimination

One of the first things owners need to realize is that dogs instinctively avoid urinating and defecating in their sleeping areas. Both urination and defecation are stimulated in dogs by eating, drinking, exercise, and excitement.

Young puppies need to eliminate frequently. They should be taken to an appropriate spot to urinate every three to four hours at first, and to defecate approximately fifteen minutes after a meal. A puppy should not be confined in a crate or cage for long periods of time or he will have no choice but to soil his sleeping area—see "Housebreaking Problems," page 39.

As a dog grows, a regular routine of walks or trips outdoors, in the morning, after eating, and so forth, will help him learn when, and where, an owner wants him to eliminate. Praise in the form of verbal encouragement or a small treat when the dog eliminates properly will also help him understand what is wanted.

Puppies of both sexes squat to urinate. As a male dog matures he will usually begin to urinate against upright objects by raising one of his rear legs. The age at which this occurs differs according to the dog's breed, size, and individual preference. Some adult males continue to squat to urinate from time to time. Adult females usually squat to urinate, but occasionally some females also lift their legs against upright objects. Even when she squats to urinate, a female dog may be marking. If she scratches the ground after urination it is marking behavior, not elimination.

Most dogs indulge in urine marking as a form of territorial behavior (see "Territorial Behavior," page 31), and some dogs will urinate small amounts as a sign of submission (see Table 2, "Canine Body Language," page 32).

Some Inappropriate Canine Behaviors

AGGRESSIVE BEHAVIOR

Aggressive behavior toward owners usually stems from what is called "dominance aggression." In other words a dog that is aggressive toward his owner is displaying his social superiority or dominance over the owner. Just as wolves in a pack vie for a dominant role, a dog may feel the need to try to dominate his owner. This type of aggression differs from territorial aggression (see page 31) in which a dog will attack a stranger who invades his property. A few dogs suffer from both types of aggression and will bite both strangers and owners.

Sometimes breeders inadvertently produce aggressive dogs by selectively breeding them for coat color, for instance, instead of for temperament. Or a breeder may be interested in developing dogs with the kind of proud, heads-up, dominant (aggressive) personalities that win dog shows, rather than for softer, nonaggressive personalities. Cocker and springer spaniels, as an example, have suffered from aggression probably because they have been bred selectively for the wrong traits. (Note: This is often wrongly referred to as "overbreeding.")

Purebred dogs in general tend to have more problems with aggression than mixed breeds. A much larger percentage of males are aggressive than females.

The best way to predict whether a puppy will turn into an aggressive dog is to meet both parents and pet them. The parents' behavior is very important. If it isn't possible to meet both parents, ask to talk to owners of pups from previous litters of the same parents or the same sire. If even one puppy from a previous litter had a problem with aggression, don't get that puppy, because this frequently is an inherited behavior in dogs.

Dogs can also be turned aggressive if they are mishandled, harshly treated, punished excessively, or teased continuously, but these dogs are more likely to be fearfully aggressive—that is, they will bite when they feel threatened.

A dog need not be aggressive to be a good watchdog. If all an owner wants is to be warned that someone is coming, a good-natured fifteen-pound terrier will make a very good watchdog. The only problem with many dogs is that they are more likely to bark at other dogs than at people (see "Excessive Barking," below). A large dog is also a very good deterrent to most burglars—the dog need not be lethally aggressive, just big.

DESTRUCTIVE BEHAVIOR

Dogs that engage in destructive behavior when their owners are away from the house are usually suffering from what is commonly called *separation anxiety.* This stems from dogs' natural social orientation system, the need to be with other pack members.

There are several forms of this misbehavior. There is what's known as *barrier frustration,* in which a dog will gouge doors and windowsills in an effort to get out. The Northern breeds of dogs such as huskies and malamutes hate to be closed up and tend to be most frequently destructive in this way. Whether their motivation to get out is to run, to find their "pack," or to have freedom, behaviorists don't know.

Separation anxiety can occur when an adult dog is left alone without his human "pack." He apparently becomes stressed and worried that perhaps he has been abandoned and will usually

aim his destructive behavior at his owner's personal possessions. Perhaps in an effort to feel close to his owner, a dog suffering from this type of anxiety will chew his human's shoes, other clothing, and so forth—items on which the owner's scent is strong.

A third type of separation anxiety seems to arise simply because of boredom. A bored dog will have no focus for his destructive activity, but will chew the edge of the sofa one day, the draperies the next, and books and magazines on yet another day.

A bored dog will benefit from extra exercise before being left alone. Distractions such as another playful dog, or a special toy that he's given only when the owner is going out, may help. Food alone usually doesn't work; the dog may be so upset he loses his appetite. But a toy with a hollow center that can be filled with soft food such as cheese will entertain many dogs for hours. Chewing also seems to relieve stress in many dogs.

In mild cases of separation anxiety confinement in a secure, dark, cavelike place such as a plastic airline kennel may help. Many dogs feel less frightened in a small space and will often reach the stage where they kennel themselves when left alone.

But a truly phobic and panic-stricken dog will need more complex help to get over his anxiety. In a case such as this, behaviorists recommend anti-anxiety medication so the dog doesn't become upset and hysterical while learning to accept being left alone.

OTHER PHOBIAS

Dogs can also suffer from a wide variety of other phobias. It's not always clear what triggers a phobia, but dogs can be terrified of such diverse stimuli as riding in the car, an open umbrella, or the smell of a certain food cooking. The most common phobia is to sudden loud noises such as thunder or gunshots, which can throw some dogs into an irrational panic in which they go through doors and even throw themselves out of upper-story windows in an effort to get away from the terrifying sound.

Desensitization with the help of a behaviorist is possible, but it is a long process that many owners are not willing to tackle. Basically, it consists of having the dog in a controlled environment and exposing him to a very mild version of whatever is frightening him while someone stays near to reward him for relaxed, nonphobic behavior. For example, a dog that is terrified of thunderstorms may hear a tape recording of thunder over and over, first at low volume, then gradually louder. His owner stays nearby and gives him a food treat if he lies quietly. This is not always successful, however, as other factors such as changes in barometric pressure or the accompanying lightning are impossible to re-create. Anti-anxiety medication is often useful to calm a dog and allow him to realize he's not going to die, while at the same time the owner is working to help him relax and accept whatever is frightening him.

Many phobias can be avoided if a puppy is exposed early in his life to a variety of different places, things, and people he doesn't know, including children of all ages. Then he will learn to accept a number of experiences and encounters as nonthreatening. This is known as *socialization*. Responsible breeders take care to socialize their puppies well, but the process needs to continue until a puppy is mature.

EXCESSIVE BARKING OR HOWLING

The Northern breeds, malamutes and huskies, for instance, may howl excessively in response to sounds such as sirens or because they are left alone.

Other domestic dogs may bark continuously when suffering from separation anxiety (see above) or simply to get their owners' attention. Dogs that are left outdoors in a yard or run all day may bark and bark at passersby, other dogs, or simply to get attention.

Although most owners want their dogs to bark to alert them to someone coming, excessive barking can become a serious problem. An indoor dog that barks excessively in the home can usually be broken of the habit by withholding the desired attention (e.g., not letting the dog out or not giving him a treat every time he barks), and saying "no" firmly when he barks. But an owner must be careful not to get into a vocal contest with a dog to see who can "bark" the loudest! For dogs that are left outdoors all day, the best cure for excessive barking is to bring them indoors.

There are various "startle" approaches that may help stop a dog from barking or howling continuously. An owner may make a loud noise, or spray the dog with water every time he barks or howls, but these steps require a vigilant owner who is always at home. A recently developed collar sprays a dog with citronella when he barks. This is an effective and nonpainful means of reprimanding the dog and teaching him not to bark when the collar is on. He can bark with impunity when the collar is off, preserving his watchdog function. In stubborn cases the help of a behaviorist may be needed.

3

HOUSEBREAKING PROBLEMS

There seems to be a big difference in breeds of dog in ease of housebreaking. Beagles, for instance, are very difficult to housebreak. At the Animal Behavior Clinic, College of Veterinary Medicine at Cornell University, a study was done to determine how easily former laboratory dogs could be house-trained in order to be successfully adopted as pets. The assumption was that the way the dogs had been housed might affect their ability to be house-trained—for instance, whether or not they had lived in cages, runs, or other forms of housing. The results were surprising. No matter how the dogs had been housed, beagles had the most difficulty learning to be housebroken. A survey covering the opinions of veterinarians and obedience judges also found that beagles and bassets were difficult to house-train. This is not to say that beagles and bassets can't be good pets.

They just take a bit more work, and easily cleaned rugs or carpets.

At the same clinic it was found that toy dogs can be hard to house-train. Perhaps because these dogs are so small, owners aren't as aware of the body language they use to indicate when they need to urinate or defecate. Most dogs let their owners know when they need to go out by sniffing around, panting, pawing, circling, scratching at the door, or something similar.

If a formerly housebroken dog suddenly starts to soil in the house, an owner must suspect a physical problem (see page 150). The first step should be to consult a veterinarian.

Barring a physical cause, housebreaking problems can be hard to solve. One solution may be the use of a crate as an aid. Because a dog doesn't want to urinate or defecate in the area in which he sleeps, this prevents a dog

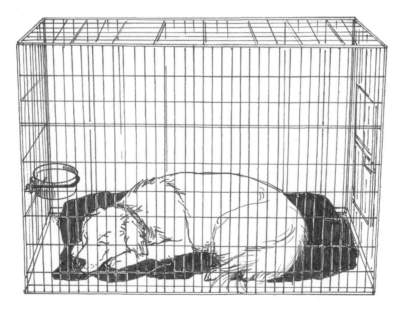

A dog in a crate. Note that the crate is large enough so that the dog can stand and move around comfortably.

from getting into the bad habit of soiling or wetting when nobody is around. If a crate is used to train a puppy, an owner must arrange for the puppy to be taken out every three hours. Otherwise the pup will have no choice but to soil or wet his crate and will learn to be a dirty dog.

PREDATORY BEHAVIOR

Predatory, or chase, behavior may sometimes be confused with territorial behavior (see page 31 for the body language that typifies chase behavior). Typically, chase behavior occurs when someone goes by a dog's property moving fast—running or riding a bicycle, for instance. The dog will immediately jump up and chase the moving person.

This is a behavior that can be easily stopped if the moving person stays still, or turns and begins to chase the dog. The dog will usually turn and run in the other direction, just as a wolf would if the moose he was chasing turned around and began running after him.

Coursing dogs such as Afghans, salukis, and greyhounds have been bred and trained to chase game by sight instead of smell. They will instinctively chase any small moving animal until they catch and kill it. Racing greyhounds are routinely rewarded for chasing rabbits or rabbit skins by being allowed to eat their prey or a food reward. So if you already own a cat, a retired racing greyhound may be a real threat to that cat and should not be considered as a pet.

ROAMING BEHAVIOR

Some dogs such as the coursing breeds (Afghans, salukis, and greyhounds) have a genetic tendency to roam. Otherwise, roaming has to have motivation. Intact (unneutered)

males roam in search of receptive females; terriers may start out running after a chipmunk and just keep going. Hounds, in general, are apt to roam—probably in search of prey.

Neutering a male dog will take away his motivation to roam in search of females. If a dog lives out in the country and his owner wants to prevent roaming, a buried electric "fence" can help. The dog wears a special collar that warns him with a "beep" before he reaches any boundary he is not supposed to cross; it then gives him a shock if he continues to advance. However, if a dog is highly motivated to roam or chase something, he may run right through the "fence." These devices are not as satisfactory in more populated areas because even if a fenced dog won't go out, other dogs can freely come and go. Electric fences should never be used for a dog that is territorially aggressive because anyone who wanders into the hidden territorial boundaries may be bitten. Otherwise, the best prevention for roaming is to keep a dog leashed and under control.

How Dogs Behave When They're Not Feeling Well

Because of their pack orientation, wolves will seek help from their pack mates, or pack leader, if they are injured or ill. A pet dog will normally come to his owner, whine, and look for help, comfort, or commiseration when he is sick or hurt. His activity level will decrease, and he may adopt a body posture that looks like a "play bow," with his hind end up in the air, front end down. This is known as the "praying" posture.

What to Do if a Behavior Problem Develops

If a dog develops a behavior problem, the first step for an owner to take is to go to the veterinarian to be sure there is no medical reason for the dog's misbehavior. For example, a housebreaking problem could be a sign of urinary tract disorder (see pages 149 to 150); sudden biting behavior might be caused by a painful ear (see pages 106 to 108), underactive thyroid, or, in the case of an older dog, a brain tumor.

Once a medical cause for the misbehavior has been ruled out, a veterinarian may be able to prescribe medication intended to modify the behavior. Or he might suggest behavior therapy and put the owner in touch with a board-certified veterinary behaviorist, or someone certified by the Animal Behavior Society, who has passed requirements and become certified to practice animal behavior. Although most dog trainers are very good at solving obedience problems, they are not behaviorists and are not qualified to treat serious behavior problems.

Owner Responsibilities

Owning a dog is a privilege, and with that privilege come responsibilities. One of those responsibilities is to make sure a pet dog doesn't infringe on or injure anyone. Leash and pooper-scooper laws, for instance, must be observed, not ignored. Because of irresponsible dog owners, many public parks now prohibit even leashed, well-trained dogs.

The other important owner responsibility is to the dog himself. Owners must take into account the fact that dogs are social animals that require companionship and entertainment on a regular basis. A person who has to be away from home fourteen hours a day, leaving a dog alone, should not own a dog. By the same token, a dog that's continuously relegated to a basement, or is tied up in a backyard all day, might as well be in a zoo. The dog will survive, but his quality of life will be very poor.

Before choosing a dog as a pet, a potential dog owner should be sure to consider the breed's particular temperament and physical care requirements, such as grooming and exercise. A pet dog should not be picked out for looks, type, or color of haircoat, but should be chosen to fit his owner's lifestyle as closely as possible in order for a successful and happy relationship to ensue.

3

NORMAL DOG BEHAVIOR

Part Two

A Sick
or Injured Dog

4

Accidents

and Medical

Emergencies

Most emergency situations involving dogs are usually due either to accidental injury or to illness. Emergencies due to accidental injury may include *trauma,* such as a bad fall, hard blow, or being hit by a moving vehicle. In these cases the dog may suffer from fractures, concussion, or other internal injuries. *Lacerations* and *wounds* can be emergency situations, especially if there is a lot of blood loss. It is an emergency situation if a dog swallows *poison* or other harmful household substances such a human medication, cleaning products, rodent poison, or even seemingly harmless foods such as chocolate. Puppies in particular can *choke* on foreign objects. A dog can be accidentally *burned, electrocuted,* or suffer from *smoke inhalation;* in rare cases, dogs can also *drown.* One of the most serious and commonly occurring emergency situations for dogs is *heat prostration.* An *illness* may be an emergency if it is sudden and acute, or an ongoing illness can become an emergency for many reasons.

Avoiding Accidents

An important thing for a dog owner to bear in mind is that no matter how smart a puppy or dog may be, she has no concept of potential danger, especially if she has lived in a protected environment all of her life. It is up to an owner to think for his pet and try to make sure she is protected from dangerous situations as far as possible.

When an owner is aware of the types of accidental emergency situations a puppy or dog can get herself into he can use his common sense to take steps to avoid them. By anticipating danger for a puppy or dog, just as he would for a human toddler, an owner can prevent many emergency situations from arising.

"Puppy-Proofing"

One of the best things the owner of a new puppy (or even an adult dog that is new to a household) can do to protect a pet from accidental injury in the home is to take time to carefully examine the space the pup will be living in, from a dog's point of view, and remove any potential hazards.

At first, it is generally best to keep a puppy or new dog in a crate or small room closed off with a pressure gate, not only for the sake of the house and furniture but to protect the pet from potential harm. At the same time, this will allow a dog to become accustomed to the household gradually. It is especially important to confine a puppy or new dog when no one will be at home to watch her.

Almost all puppies will chew anything they can to help relieve boredom or the discomfort of teething. Chewing is also used by dogs as a means of exploration. Small objects such as pencils, toys, bones, and other items that can be chewed into small pieces and swallowed should never be left in an area where a puppy can reach them. If they are chewed and swallowed the puppy may *choke,* or the pieces can become lodged in the pup's esophagus. If so, they will have to be removed by a veterinarian. Objects that are sharp or hard may injure a dog's throat.

Puppies will also chew electric wires if they are within reach. If the wires are plugged in, a pup can easily be *electrocuted.* Even if wires are not plugged in, a curious puppy may pull a dangling wire and be injured by a falling lamp or appliance.

Trauma

Trauma from a dog's being hit by a car, motorcycle, or bicycle can usually be avoided by keeping a puppy or dog under control whenever she is outdoors. If she is in an enclosed yard or run, an owner must be sure the gate or door to the enclosure is securely closed and latched—a loosely latched gate can easily be pushed open by an excited pup, anxious to get out and play with another dog or children who are passing by. Out of the yard a dog needs to be securely leashed. It's important to make certain whatever type of collar is used cannot accidentally slip off over a dog's head if she tries to pull away.

When riding in a car a dog should always be crated or securely leashed so she cannot jump out of a suddenly opened door or window. Another danger can occur if a puppy or dog tries to bolt out the front door of the house when it's opened. If a dog shows a tendency to do this she ought to be held or confined whenever the door is opened, until she can be trained not to run out into the street.

Puppies can also suffer from trauma when

they fall from windows. The term *high-rise syndrome* is usually associated with kittens and cats that live in apartments in cities, but puppies, too, frequently fall from open windows. Puppies are just as lacking in judgment as kittens, and just as curious, and they may lean too far out a window and lose their balance very quickly. A pup need not fall far to hurt herself badly. A fall from a second-story window onto a flagstone path or tiled terrace can be just as damaging as one from a fourth-floor apartment window. Never leave a puppy alone in a room with an open, unscreened window. The most sensible safety measures are either to open windows only from the top, or make certain they have secure screens until the puppy grows up a bit and develops some judgment.

Poisoning

Accidental poisoning is a very common canine emergency. Curious puppies are the most frequent victims, but because many adult dogs will usually eat just about anything vaguely resembling food, they are also often poisoned.

Many common household chemicals are poisonous to dogs as well as humans, but most do not appeal to dogs because of their foul smell or taste. An exception to this is *antifreeze,* which has a sweetish taste that is irresistible to dogs. Antifreeze contains ethylene glycol, which is highly toxic and can be fatal to dogs. Antifreeze should be kept in tightly closed containers and extreme care needs to be taken that no radiator fluid containing antifreeze has leaked onto a driveway or garage floor. This is especially important if a normally outdoor dog is put in a garage to sleep at night during cold weather. A dog that is suspected of ingesting antifreeze

needs *immediate* veterinary care to prevent kidney failure and eventual death. There is now a safer antifreeze on the market that is propylene glycol, rather than ethylene glycol.

Rat poison is another insidious danger for dogs. It is designed to be attractive to animals and is often packaged in tasty, good-smelling suet cakes, which dogs will readily eat. Rat poisons contain a substance called warfarin, or similar chemicals, that interfere with a dog's blood-clotting ability and blocks the production of vitamin K. A dog that has eaten rat poison may become anemic, have trouble breathing, suffer from nosebleeds, internal bleeding, and bruising. Prompt treatment with vitamin K injections and blood transfusions will usually help.

Human medications and recreational drugs can cause severe *drug intoxication* in dogs and ought to be kept out of their reach. Owners need to realize that *no* medication is safe to give to a dog except on the advice of a veterinarian.

Alcohol and *nicotine* can make dogs very sick, as can many kinds of "people food," because they are too rich for dogs. As we explained on page 22, *chocolate* is especially toxic.

Although warnings about *plant poisoning* are issued annually, usually around holiday times, such poisoning is rare with dogs because they don't often chew plant leaves.

Dog owners were warned for years about the poisonous nature of poinsettias. But in 1989 it was reported in many veterinary medical journals that a pharmacist affiliated with the Hennipin Regional Poison Center in Minneapolis uncovered studies that showed not a single published report of poinsettia toxicity in dogs had been seen since 1919. However, the sap from some holiday plants and berries, such as holly and mistletoe make a dog ill. Japanese yew can be fatal to dogs and ingestion of dieffenbachia (dumbcane) can cause painful and potentially dangerous swelling of the mucous membranes of a dog's mouth and throat.

If a puppy or dog is known to have eaten anything potentially poisonous, the owner should immediately call a veterinarian. If a veterinarian cannot be reached, call the ASPCA National Animal Poison Control Center at 800-548-2423. This center is manned by veterinarians and board-certified toxicologists and is open twenty-four hours a day, every day. A $30 consultation fee is payable by credit card. If possible, the owner should have information available about the substance ingested. Immediate action can often prevent permanent health damage and even death.

For free nonemergency information about pesticides concerning both animals and people, call the National Pesticide Telecommunications Network (NPTN) at 800-858-7378. At this number, graduate scientists will answer inquiries about lawn-care and gardening products, pest-control products, and so forth as they might affect both pets and people. This service, available from 6:30 A.M. to 4:30 P.M. Pacific time, seven days a week, excluding holidays, is a cooperative effort of Oregon State University and the U.S. Environmental Protection Agency. See also "Drug Poisoning/Intoxication," on page 55, and Appendix A, page 157.

Heat Prostration

The most common reason dogs suffer from heat prostration is because they are left in parked cars during hot weather. On a moderate, sunny day when the temperature is in the seventies, it takes only a few minutes of sunshine on a car for the interior to heat up to over a hundred degrees, even if the windows are partially open. Because a dog has no way to cool her body other than panting, which is not very efficient, she will quickly collapse in an ovenlike car. It's a serious mistake to think that parking in a shady spot will protect a dog, because the sun can move very quickly, turning a shady spot sunny. The best prevention for this serious emergency is to leave a dog at home on warm days.

If a dog does appear to have difficulty breathing, or collapses from the heat, she must be rushed to a veterinarian immediately in order to save her life. More about heat prostration can be found on pages 55 to 56.

Some Canine Medical Emergencies

As we said above, an ongoing illness can develop into an emergency for various reasons. A severe medical problem that occurs suddenly is also an emergency situation. Following are some commonly occurring medical emergencies. In most instances there are no effective home first aid steps that can be taken, and prompt veterinary care is necessary.

Bleeding Internally

BLOODY DIARRHEA OR STOOL

When a dog is passing normal stools or diarrhea containing small specks or streaks of blood, there is no severe emergency; however, a veterinarian should be consulted during normal office hours. On the other hand, if bleeding is profuse and the dog is producing only pools of dark, foul-smelling blood, she may be suffering from *hemorrhagic gastroenteritis* (HGE) (see page 102), a severe, life-threatening emergency, especially for small dogs, which may go into shock (see Box, page 53) within hours. Because this type of bloody diarrhea contains a great deal of water, the fluid loss can lead to a specific kind of shock, called *hypovolemic shock*. Immediate veterinary treatment is essential; there is no first aid for serious blood loss in the stool.

BLOOD IN THE URINE

Bloody urine usually signifies some type of urinary tract or bladder infection (see page 52), and although veterinary treatment is needed, it is not a serious medical emergency. Sometimes it is accompanied by straining to urinate and/or passing only small amounts of urine. If, however, blood clots are present, or the urine becomes very dark red in color, it indicates severe bleeding in the urinary tract. This requires immediate veterinary treatment. As above, there is no first aid for serious blood loss in the urine.

VOMITING BLOOD

If a dog vomits fluid containing flecks or streaks of blood it is not a serious emergency. But if a large amount of blood is thrown up, or blood clots are contained in the vomitus, it can be a sign of significant internal bleeding. There is no first aid for this condition, which requires immediate veterinary attention. Oral medications should *not* be given when a dog is vomiting blood.

SPONTANEOUS BRUISING

Bruising can be difficult for an owner to recognize because of a dog's haircoat. If there are purple splotches on a dog's stomach it can be a sign of a bleeding disorder. If an owner sees little purple or red spots on a dog's gums or the insides of her ears, it can be because of a low platelet count (thrombocytopenia), or another kind of bleeding disorder. In some cases a dog can bleed

into internal cavities such as the chest, abdomen, or the brain, which can cause severe problems. Bruising of any sort should be considered serious, and veterinary care sought.

Bloat (see "Gastric Dilatation/ Volvulus [GDV] Complex," below)

Breathing Problems

Breathing problems are usually caused by fluid in the lungs, in the chest area around the lungs, or because of air in a dog's chest cavity (pneumothorax). A dog with breathing problems will seem to be breathing deeply in an effort to get enough oxygen, and she may have purple or bluish mucous membranes (cyanosis).

If a dog has difficulty breathing it can be caused by several conditions: a traumatic chest injury, congestive heart failure (see below), or serious pneumonia (see "Respiratory Difficulties," pages 136 to 139). It is always a severe emergency requiring immediate veterinary care.

Cardiovascular Emergencies

CONGESTIVE HEART FAILURE

This condition most commonly occurs in older small or toy breeds of dog. Usually there have been some previous symptoms of a problem, such as a chronic cough at night when the dog is quiet. (Note: Small dogs may also suffer from collapsed tracheas [see pages 115 and 138], which causes them to cough. In this case, however, they generally cough when they are active, not at night when they are quiet.) The lungs of a dog with this condition will have filled with water (pulmonary edema), allowing very little oxygen to be absorbed into the bloodstream, which causes the dog to have considerable difficulty breathing. She will either breathe rapidly in gasps, or seem to suck air into her stomach; her abdomen will move in and out visibly each time she takes a breath. At this point it is essential to keep the dog quiet and calm and get her to the veterinarian as soon as possible. If she becomes stressed or excited it might cause her to collapse or suffer cardiac arrest. A dog in this condition may have purple or bluish mucous membranes (the gums and insides of her mouth). This is a very serious condition known as *cyanosis,* and signifies a severe lack of oxygen in the bloodstream.

IRREGULAR HEARTBEAT (CARDIAC ARRHYTHMIA)

A dog with a significantly irregular heartbeat will seem to be in shock (see Box, page 53). She will be confused and weak and may collapse. The mucous membranes in her mouth will be pale pink to white because her heart is not circulating her blood properly. This can be due to a serious increase of the heart rate above normal, called *tachycardia,* or to a severe slowing of the heart rate, called *bradycardia.* Both conditions are serious emergencies. The dog should be kept quiet and stress free, and immediate veterinary care sought.

Collapse

Collapse, sometimes accompanied by unconsciousness, can be due to a number of medical conditions described in this chapter, such as congestive heart failure, heart arrhythmias, hypoglycemia, shock, and heat prostration. It can also be caused by a severe trauma, hypoxia (poor oxygenation), or blood loss. Sometimes it is because

of an undetected internal condition, such as a ruptured tumor (hemangiosarcoma), or severe infection that has caused the dog to become weak. Seizures, serious muscle disorders, and electrolyte problems can also cause a dog to collapse. It is an extremely serious symptom, the cause of which must be diagnosed and treated quickly.

Diarrhea

Diarrhea is fairly common in dogs and usually does not constitute a medical emergency. Exceptions are if the diarrhea contains quantities of blood (see "Bloody Diarrhea or Stool," above); is explosive; lasts for more than twenty-four hours; or is accompanied by other symptoms such as vomiting, loss of appetite, and signs of pain or illness such as listlessness or depression. In these cases it can be a symptom of poisoning (see pages 47 to 48), a systemic illness, or a serious infectious disease such as distemper (see page 58) or parvovirus (see page 58). See also pages 101 to 105.

Gastric Dilatation/Volvulus (GDV) Complex—"Bloat"

This is a condition that occurs most frequently in large, deep-chested dogs that weigh over fifty pounds. The dog's stomach expands and fills with gas, which puts pressure on all the internal organs, including the diaphragm and large blood vessels, and prevents proper breathing and blood circulation. Initial signs include frequent, ineffective attempts by the dog to retch and vomit, enlargement of the abdomen, and difficulty breathing, followed by confusion, weakness, and eventual shock and collapse. This is an extremely serious condition and immediate veterinary intervention is needed in order to save the dog.

Hypoglycemia

Hypoglycemia, or low blood sugar, is characterized by several different signs. A dog with this condition may be weak and confused. She may not respond to her name, and will pace or wander aimlessly at first. Signs of weakness will usually occur first in the hind legs and move on to the front limbs. Eventually the dog will be unable to stand. During this time she will retain consciousness but as time passes, she may go into a coma (unconscious, unresponsive state).

Another form of the disorder is the sudden onset of *seizures* or *convulsions*. During a seizure, a dog will lie on her side and move her jaws rapidly while producing a great deal of saliva. She will involuntarily produce urine and feces, shake or "paddle" her limbs violently, and eventually lapse into a coma. Even with proper treatment, brain damage may occur.

Hypoglycemia occurs for several reasons. When small-breed puppies, especially Yorkshire terriers, go without eating for even short periods of time, they can quickly become hypoglycemic. Dogs with diabetes mellitus that are on insulin treatment can develop hypoglycemia if the proper food and insulin balance is not maintained. Sometimes older dogs suffer from insulin-producing pancreatic tumors, which can cause hypoglycemia.

With hypoglycemia, first aid treatment can help. Honey, syrup, or sugar water may reverse the problem for a puppy that begins to become confused or weak due to lack of eating properly, but only if it is given at the first signs of a prob-

lem, before collapse or seizures occur. If a diabetic dog that has had too much insulin and shows signs of weakness is given sugar promptly, it can prevent further problems from developing; the same is true for older dogs with insulin-producing tumors. Dosage depends on the size of the dog. Approximately a tablespoon given a little at a time is probably enough for a small dog, more if a dog is larger. Do not attempt to give anything orally if a dog is unconscious. A veterinary checkup should be given once the dog is stabilized.

Pyometra

This is a severe infection of the uterus that occurs usually in middle-aged or older unspayed female dogs, often several weeks after a heat cycle has ended. A dog with a pyometra will be very sick. She will lose her appetite, vomit, have diarrhea, may run a fever, have increased thirst and excessive urination. Immediate surgical removal of the uterus is the treatment of choice. See also Box, page 113.

Seizures/Convulsions

Seizures in dogs can be due to a medical condition such as hypoglycemia (see above) or canine distemper in puppies. They can also be caused by idiopathic epilepsy (of no known cause), which usually surfaces when a dog is one to three years old.

A seizure can be mild and take the form of a moment or two of lost consciousness, or it may be violent and severe and last up to several minutes. There is a description of a violent seizure above, under "Hypoglycemia." After a violent seizure there is often what is called a postictal period, when the dog is quiet and still, pants or breathes fast, and then slowly comes back to normal.

If a seizure is short and the dog then returns to normal, it is not a serious emergency. However, if a dog has several continuous seizures that last a long time (status epilecticus), she may die or have permanent brain damage due to hypoxia (a loss of oxygen in the tissues).

There is nothing an owner can do to help a dog having a seizure except to protect her from harming herself. The myth that dogs may swallow their tongues during a seizure is not true, and an owner who tries to intervene by putting his hand in a dog's mouth can be bitten involuntarily by the dog in the midst of a seizure. The dog should be placed on the floor on her side and the area cleared of objects that could fall on the dog.

Veterinary assessment and treatment are necessary for any dog that has suffered from a seizure. An owner's observations about the seizure—its onset, length, severity, and any other details he can remember—will provide the veterinarian with the information he needs in order to properly treat the dog.

Spinal Problems

An acute onset of trouble with both rear legs is often a sign that a dog is suffering from some type of spinal problem. In a severe case a dog will cry out in pain and her rear legs will collapse. If the damage is less severe, the dog may seem to have pain and discomfort but is still able to walk, although her back legs may not seem to work well.

Ruptured, or slipped, spinal discs (invertebral disc disease) most often occur in long-bodied dogs such as dachshunds and basset hounds, or in small or toy dogs. There is nothing an owner can do to relieve this problem. Immediate veterinary help is needed, but even with prompt medical attention it is possible for the spinal cord to suffer from irreparable damage, resulting in paralysis of the rear legs. See also pages 117 to 118.

Splenic Tumor, Ruptured

A dog with a ruptured tumor (hemangiosarcoma) of the spleen or liver will be in shock (see Box, opposite). Her mucous membranes will be pale and she will be weak and may collapse. Sometimes there will be no sign of this condition except a swollen abdomen and lethargy. This is a condition needing immediate veterinary attention. It is seen most often in large dogs, especially retrievers and German shepherds.

Unconsciousness (see "Collapse," page 50)

Urinary Emergencies

A dog with a bacterial infection of the bladder (cystitis) will feel as if she has a full bladder all the time, and will attempt to urinate often (pollakiuria) while producing only small amounts of urine each time. A dog with this condition will usually seem to feel well and will not lose her appetite. Although this is not an emergency, it should be treated promptly to relieve the dog's discomfort. On the other hand, a dog with an obstruction in her urinary tract such as a urinary tract stone will attempt to urinate frequently but will not be able to pass any urine. A dog with this

Shock

When a dog is injured or is suffering from a severe medical emergency, she may be in a condition known as shock, in which her cardiovascular system collapses. This means that the body's tissues are not being properly oxygenated due to inadequate blood circulation. Symptoms of shock are: physical weakness and collapse; confusion; shivering; a weak, rapid pulse; rapid heartbeat; and pale mucous membranes, which can be observed by looking in the dog's mouth. Normally, a dog's gums and the insides of her cheeks are bright pink. If her mucous membranes are pale pink she is in mild shock or anemic; if they are white, her condition is extremely serious. If shock has been brought about by heavy blood loss, it is called *hemorrhagic shock*. Serious body water loss can lead to *hypovolemic shock*.

A dog suspected of being in shock should be kept warm and quiet and have immediate veterinary care, including intravenous fluids. If shock is not treated promptly and aggressively, a dog will die.

problem will seem sick, lose her appetite, and may vomit. This is an emergency that requires immediate veterinary care. See also "Blood in the Urine," page 49.

Vomiting

If a dog vomits but seems to feel well otherwise, it is usually not an emergency. But if a dog vomits for more than twenty-four hours, or vomits more than 4 to 5 times in a day on an empty stomach, there is blood in the vomitus (see "Vomiting Blood," page 49), or the dog has other symptoms such as diarrhea, loss of appetite, weakness, abdominal swelling, or other signs of illness, it may be an indication of a serious medical condition requiring immediate veterinary action such as pancreatitis, intestinal blockage, kidney, or liver problems. See also: "Gastric Dilatation/Volvulus (GDV) Complex," "Poisoning," and "Shock" in this chapter.

Whelping Emergencies

DYSTOCIA

If more than four hours go by without a puppy appearing while a dog is still in labor, or more than two hours between puppies, the mother is probably suffering from dystocia. A mother dog in labor who suddenly becomes weak and stops pushing is also experiencing dystocia. In either instance, without veterinary intervention, the puppy will die and the mother dog may develop medical problems as well.

ECLAMPSIA OR HYPOCALCEMIA

Toy breeds (Chihuahuas, toy poodles, Yorkshire terriers) most often suffer from this problem, especially when they have large litters of puppies. It usually occurs after birth when the puppies have nursed for a while, but it can surface before whelping. It is caused by a rapid drop in the mother's blood calcium level because of the excessive calcium demand both before birth and during nursing. Symptoms are excessive panting, fever, trembling, shaking, and possible collapse. This condition requires immediate intravenous calcium to prevent central nervous system damage and even coma or death.

Some Accidental Canine Emergencies

In general, the best treatment an owner can provide for a pet suffering from an accidental injury is to get her to a veterinarian right away. It is foolish and dangerous to waste precious time trying to give emergency first aid, and often whatever measures that are taken won't help and may harm a dog. If there are first aid steps that may be helpful they are included here.

Bleeding

Bleeding from any part of a dog's body is an emergency if there is a great deal of blood loss or if slow bleeding continues for any length of time. The best way to determine if the bleeding is serious is to check the dog for any signs of shock (see Box, page 53).

BLEEDING FROM THE NOSE OR MOUTH

This can be life-threatening if there is a lot of blood. Cold compresses or ice packs can slow the bleeding but are very difficult to apply. The best treatment is to get a dog to a veterinarian immediately.

BLEEDING FROM THE SKIN

Cuts or wounds on a dog's skin surface will cause some bleeding although it is usually not severe. If a wound is deep it can puncture a vein or blood vessel beneath the skin surface and bleeding will be more profuse. This happens most often in dogs if the wound is in the neck or leg area (see below). Pressure should be applied to slow the bleeding, either with a clean cloth or by hand if the area is difficult to bandage. (See illustration of a compression, or pressure, bandage in Chapter 6, page 68.)

FOOT AND LEG BLEEDING

Dogs' footpads bleed a great deal when they are cut. The pads consist of spongelike tissue, and cuts will open up and continue to bleed each time a dog puts her weight on her foot. To prevent continuous blood loss from a footpad laceration, a pressure bandage should be used, held in place with a sock if necessary (see illustration, page 68).

More serious, spurting, arterial bleeding can occur if a dog cuts the small artery that runs up the leg right behind the footpads—a very common injury. This type of bleeding should be stopped with a pressure bandage placed around the entire foot. Again, a sock placed over the bandage will help hold it in place but care must be taken not to tie anything tight around the dog's leg that will cut off the circulation in the foot. *The use of tourniquets is not advised.* They can easily cause the loss of a limb due to inadequate blood supply and do not stop bleeding as well as pressure.

If there is bleeding higher up on a dog's leg it also should be treated with a compression bandage.

Broken Bones

A dog can break any one of the hundreds of bones in her body, but the most common canine fractures are those of the legs and feet. A dog with a broken limb should be kept quiet, treated for shock (see Box, page 53), and moved as little as possible. A makeshift stretcher for a large dog, or cardboard box or board for a smaller animal, will prevent the injured limb from moving around while the dog is transported to the veterinarian (see "Transporting an Injured Dog," pages 67 to 68). Splints or other ways of immobilizing an injured limb are not recommended for dogs.

Burns

A dog can burn her throat and/or esophagus if she swallows overheated food. A veterinarian should be consulted in case the damage to the dog's throat is severe. A damaged esophagus can scar, causing a narrowing or stricture, which will make eating or drinking impossible.

A dog can be seriously burned if scalding water or hot grease falls on her or if she falls into a tub of scalding water. This is a serious emergency and prompt veterinary care is critical. As with humans, a serious burn over a large part of the body can be fatal.

Drug Poisoning/Intoxication

Almost any human medicine can poison a dog, as can drugs such as marijuana, hashish, hallucinogenics, and so forth. If an owner knows that a dog has ingested medication or drugs that are not caustic, he should get the material out of the dog quickly by inducing vomiting. One to two teaspoons of Ipecac or hydrogen peroxide (1:1 with water) given orally with a spoon will cause a dog to vomit and will not harm the dog. The dog should be seen by a veterinarian right away to be sure no drug remains in her body and

to check for any side effects. See also "Poisoning," pages 47 to 48, and Appendix A, page 157.

Electrocution

As we mentioned earlier, puppies are more apt to suffer from electrocution than adult dogs because of their tendency to chew on anything, including plugged-in electric wires. If an owner comes home and finds a puppy with a plugged-in electric cord still in her mouth, he should be very careful to unplug the cord before touching the puppy! If a puppy is lying on her side, unable to move and having trouble breathing, he should realize the puppy has probably bitten a wire and has been electrocuted. If the puppy appears to be in shock (see Box, page 53) or exhibits signs of cyanosis (blue mucous membranes), it is probably an indication that she has fluid in her lungs from electrocution. This is a serious emergency requiring immediate veterinary help.

Eye Injuries

Although the brachycephalic breeds of dogs with protruding, unprotected eyes frequently suffer from eye injuries, other dog breeds may also injure their eyes. If a dog's eyeball bulges out of its socket, it is a serious emergency because if the eyeball dries out, it may not be possible to save the eye. No first aid, such as putting water on the eye, should be attempted as it will upset the delicate eye membranes and will do more harm than good.

Heat Prostration

We spoke about heat prostration earlier in this chapter. Although it occurs most often when a dog is left in a closed car in warm weather, it can also affect a dog that is closed in a hot, airless room. Any dog that regularly has a difficult time breathing, such as an extremely brachycephalic dog, a severely overweight animal, or one with a heart condition, may suffer from heat prostration if she becomes overheated or overexerts.

Contagious

and

Infectious

Diseases

Dogs are susceptible to a number of infectious and contagious diseases, just like all mammals. Infectious diseases are caused when a dog's body is invaded by a disease-producing entity or entities such as bacteria, fungi, protozoa, parasites, or viruses. Contagious diseases are infectious diseases that can be passed from one dog to another. Thus, contagious diseases are always infectious, but not all infectious diseases are contagious (that is, able to be "caught" by a dog from another dog). In general, bacterial diseases are less contagious than viral diseases, which are usually very contagious.

Contagious diseases can be transmitted from one dog to another by various means. These include direct contact with an infected dog or with his urine, feces, saliva, or blood, or the inhaling of airborne viruses or bacteria, which does not require direct contact between dogs. Some infectious diseases are transmitted by an intermediate host such as an insect or parasite that moves from a diseased animal to a well one, carrying the disease.

Fortunately, routine immunizations are almost entirely able to prevent the majority of canine infectious viral diseases. Most parasitic diseases can also be avoided by the use of preventive medications given on a schedule provided by the veterinarian. Diseases that cannot be prevented can usually be successfully treated nowadays, providing treatment is begun as soon as symptoms appear.

Infectious Viral Diseases Against Which Dogs Can Be Immunized

CANINE DISTEMPER

Canine distemper is a highly contagious viral disease that usually affects puppies but can occur in older dogs. It begins with coldlike symptoms, including runny eyes, fever, listlessness, and a runny nose. These signs may be accompanied by vomiting and diarrhea. In a short period of time, the "cold" becomes worse and a pup develops heavy nose and eye discharges, a cough, possible involuntary neurological twitching, and seizures. Once a dog has been exposed the incubation period of the disease ranges from two days to two weeks. Diagnosis is made based primarily on history and symptoms.

Once a dog has developed distemper the only treatment is to give supportive care to help the dog's body fight the disease, such as intravenous fluids and antibiotics, which may also help prevent secondary infections from occurring. While it is possible for a dog to survive distemper, the mortality rate is high; once neurologic signs occur, they may be permanent even if the dog survives.

This disease, once fatal to many puppies, has become much less common because of proper immunizations. However, as we pointed out in Chapter 2, it is important that a puppy receive the full series of vaccinations, because the first vaccines in the series may fail to protect the puppy from distemper. This is one reason why it is so important to have a veterinarian see a new puppy or dog as soon as possible so that effective immunizations can begin.

INFECTIOUS CANINE HEPATITIS

This is a viral disease that is not often seen because dogs are normally given protective vaccinations. However, young puppies that have not been immunized against this disease may become victims. Canine hepatitis is often mistakenly diagnosed as canine distemper because the symptoms are similar.

Canine hepatitis is spread by direct contact with an infected individual. The virus settles in a dog's tonsils, from where it travels through the bloodstream, lodging primarily in the kidneys and liver.

Young puppies with infectious canine hepatitis rarely survive, despite hospitalization and supportive treatment.

CANINE PARVOVIRUS

Canine parvovirus, or "parvo," is another highly contagious canine viral disease, one that caused a worldwide epidemic among domestic dogs in the late 1970s. The symptoms of parvovirus are gastrointestinal and include vomiting, bloody diarrhea, fever, and severe abdominal discomfort. The symptoms usually come on suddenly, but an owner may notice some appetite loss for a day or two before other symptoms surface. The incubation period of parvovirus is three to twelve days. An untreated affected dog can die within days of onset of the disease from dehydration, shock, or septicemia (bacterial infection in the bloodstream). Septicemia may occur because the virus suppresses the body's ability to make white blood cells. Diagnosis is made by a combination of clinical signs, history, and laboratory tests, in particular a stool test to identify the virus and a complete blood count to demonstrate a low white blood count (leukopenia).

Parvovirus is usually spread by direct contact with the feces of an infected dog, or when the feces is carried on the shoes or clothing of people. This is a very stable virus and may persist in the environment for years. Although antibiotics are not directly effective against this viral disease, they are routinely given to prevent secondary bacterial infections. Intravenous fluid therapy, supportive care, and withholding of food and water are also included in the treatment. As with canine distemper, early diagnosis and treatment are essential for success in this often fatal disease.

There is a vaccine against canine parvovirus, which should be part of every puppy's and dog's routine immunizations (see pages 17 and 18). Chlorine bleach has been found to destroy the virus and should be used in solution (1 part bleach to 9 parts water) to clean kennels, veterinary hospitals, grooming establishments, and any other areas where dogs are regularly in close proximity.

RABIES

This ancient, fatal viral disease occurs throughout the world. It is primarily transmitted in the saliva of an animal affected with the disease, which is why animal bites are viewed with suspicion. Once rabies is contracted there is no cure. The incubation period of rabies varies tremendously and can range anywhere from one week up to a year. It has been shown that an infected animal will die from rabies within ten days of the virus appearing in his saliva. Therefore, animals who bite humans should be observed for signs of illness for ten days after the bite.

The symptoms vary but almost always consist of strange, uncharacteristic behavior, either a dog who is very subdued or one who is wildly aggressive. Other signs include neurologic disease, paralysis of a limb or limbs, and difficulty swallowing.

Vaccination against rabies, followed by regular "booster" shots (see Chapter 2), is vital for all pet dogs.

"KENNEL COUGH," OR CANINE INFECTIOUS TRACHEOBRONCHITIS

This is a highly contagious condition, with both viral (parainfluenza) and bacterial (bordatella) factors. It is spread in the air and is more of a problem in areas with poor air circulation. Stress is also thought to contribute to a dog's susceptibility to the disease. It is characterized by a harsh, honking cough that is made worse if the dog pulls against his collar. It always occurs after a dog has been in close contact with other dogs, such as in a boarding kennel, hence the name. Symptoms usually appear about a week after exposure.

The disease is not serious and often goes away by itself, but if it persists or bothers the dog, cough suppressants and antibiotics may be given. Kennel cough can be prevented with injectable parainfluenza vaccine, which is usually included with distemper and hepatitis vaccines. A new bordatella vaccine, which is administered directly into the nose, seems to be more effective than the parainfluenza vaccine. Many kennels now require all dogs to have vaccinations against kennel cough before accepting them for boarding.

Fungal Canine Diseases

In addition to ringworm (see page 63), there are several other canine fungal diseases.

Aspergillosis is a fungus that usually attacks the respiratory tract of dogs. It is found in the air, the soil, moldy animal feeds, and decaying hay or vegetable matter. An affected dog will have either unilateral or bilateral watery, sometimes bloody nasal discharge, possible nosebleeds, and nasal ulcers. German shepherds and collies are frequently affected. Diagnosis can be difficult, and may include X rays, laboratory tests, biopsy, and possible surgery to inspect damage. Treatment usually consists of a combination of oral antifungal medication and flushing of the nasal passages with antifungal medication. Treatment may continue for up to two months.

There are four *mycoses,* which are fairly uncommon but are serious in the dog. These fungal diseases are usually contracted by inhalation, or possibly punctures through the skin, and then spread to the animal's internal organs or other tissues. The fungi that cause these diseases usually prefer particular environments and, therefore, are limited to specific geographic locations.

Blastomycosis is found in the soil in the north-central states, the Ohio-Mississippi river valleys, and the mid-Atlantic states. Signs of an infection are numerous and may include: eye disease, central nervous system irregularities, respiratory disease, and bone, lymph node, or skin lesions. Diagnosis is made through biopsy and microscopic examination of tissue. Treatment is with long-term systemic antifungal medication.

Histoplasmosis is also a soil fungus. It prefers humid, moist soil, contaminated by bat, wild bird, and especially chicken droppings. It is common in the Midwest and East. It is characterized by low fever, lethargy, and cough, or there may be no external signs of an infection. It may spread throughout the lungs, causing pneumonia, or to the gastrointestinal tract, producing chronic, watery diarrhea. It can also progress to the liver, spleen, or bone marrow, and may produce jaundice, or an accumulation of fluid in the abdominal area (ascites). Diagnosis is made by biopsy, and treatment is with antifungal medication, given for up to six months.

Coccidioidomycosis is the most serious of the mycoses. It is found in dry, desert areas where the creosote bush grows (central Texas to California) and can affect both dogs and humans, but is not contagious. In most dogs it affects the lungs, but in a few it may spread to eyes, bones and joints, liver, and kidneys. If it enters a dog's body through a break in the skin, it is usually localized. Diagnosis is made by microscopic examination of biopsied material, and antifungal medication must be given for a year or more.

Cryptococcosis is found in bird droppings, especially that of pigeons, and in soil contaminated by them. It attacks the central nervous system and seems to prefer young, large-breed dogs. Signs are mostly neurologic and include circling, disorientation, head tilt, incoordination, seizures, and possible paralysis. Diagnosis is made with specialized tests or biopsy. Treatment is difficult, because the disease is not always responsive to antifungal medication due to the fact that it attacks the central nervous system.

Parasitic Canine Diseases

Blood-borne parasitic canine diseases are not contagious in the usual sense, but are spread by ingestion of infectious eggs or larvae or through an intermediate host such as a mosquito, flea, or tick, which bites an infected animal and then bites an uninfected dog, depositing the disease organisms into his bloodstream.

CANINE EHRLICHIOSIS

Spread primarily by the brown dog tick, this is a disease that affects a dog's lymph nodes, spleen, liver, and blood cells. It occurs most commonly in tropical and semitropical areas, but has been seen worldwide wherever the brown tick is found. The disease is becoming much more common in the United States. It is caused by a virus-like organism classified as *Rickettsia.*

The disease usually goes through an acute stage and then may progress to a chronic condition. During the acute part of the disease a dog will exhibit fever, lack of appetite, stiffness, some eye and nasal discharge, and mild lymph node swelling. There is a drop in blood platelet levels. This stage of the disease, diagnosed by a combination of clinical signs and blood tests, usually lasts anywhere from two to four weeks. Early treatment with appropriate antibiotics is usually successful.

If the disease passes on to a chronic condition, a dog's blood cell production within the bone marrow is severely compromised and may lead to bloody stools, bloody nose, and urine. This stage lasts for months, during which time an affected dog requires continuous monitoring and therapy.

There is no preventive vaccination against ehrlichiosis.

HEARTWORM DISEASE

As its name indicates, this is a disease that affects a dog's heart. It is carried by mosquitoes, which bite an infected dog, ingest immature worm larvae, and then deposit the immature worm larvae into the skin and bloodstream of another, uninfected dog. After they develop, the infective larvae migrate into a dog's heart and large blood vessels, where they can grow to enormous lengths and, if left untreated, will eventually cause severe heart and lung problems and death.

Symptoms of heartworm disease are similar to those of other cardiac diseases (see page 49), such as lack of energy, listlessness, appetite loss, and coughing. Diagnosis is made by a blood test given prior to the mosquito season, which varies in different parts of the country. A dog that is found to be free of heartworms should be given medication to prevent contraction of the disease if he is bitten by a carrier mosquito. There are now chewable tablets that can be given once a month, but the form and timing of prevention may vary according to climate and geographic location.

If the blood test shows that a dog has already contracted heartworm disease, the dog must be treated to kill the heartworm. This treatment is difficult and some dogs will die from or during the treatment. Recovery is usually over several months and some damage may be irreversible. For this reason, prevention is strongly advised.

LYME DISEASE

Depending on the region of the country, different tick species are the carriers of Lyme disease, a bacterial disease that affects the joints of both humans and dogs, as well as those of other mammals. It is most commonly found in the northeastern and midwestern states. In contrast to the progression of the disease in humans, who may suffer from chronic pain, it is apt to take a more acute form in dogs and is usually successfully treated in the acute stage.

Symptoms of Lyme disease in dogs are varied and may include a sudden onset of lameness, joint pain, fever, enlarged lymph nodes, and loss of appetite. If a dog is known to have been bitten by a tick, early treatment may prevent further symptoms. It is diagnosed by a series of blood tests and can be treated with antibiotics.

Although the first vaccine developed for Lyme disease caused many side effects, some lethal, a safer vaccine made by use of recombinant DNA technology has now been developed and is given in areas where the incidence of the disease is high. A veterinarian can best decide when it is appropriate to give the vaccine.

ROCKY MOUNTAIN SPOTTED FEVER

Rocky Mountain spotted fever is another Rickettsial disease spread by ticks, particularly the wood tick in the West and the American dog tick in eastern states. Contrary to its name, the disease can occur anywhere, but is most prevalent in the forested areas of the mid-Atlantic states and Northeast. This disease usually surfaces in early spring to late fall, when ticks are active and feeding.

The disease attacks a dog's lymphatic system and blood vessels. Initial symptoms include appetite loss, fever, depression, lethargy, vomiting, diarrhea, and mild coldlike symptoms. Some dogs will completely recover from this stage. If the disease progresses it may produce swelling of

the limbs, facial area, ears, and scrotum. Hemorrhaging may occur in a dog's mucous membranes. Damage to all parts of a dog's body due to loss of blood supply can include tissue death, eye abnormalities, and various neurologic signs such as confusion, lack of coordination, and even coma.

Diagnosis is made by laboratory test, observation, and according to the dog's history and the time of year. Despite its name, derived from a characteristic rash in humans, the rash is usually not evident in dogs. Treatment includes antibiotics and supportive care. The prognosis for recovery is good when a dog is treated in the early stages of the disease.

There is no preventive vaccine for Rocky Mountain spotted fever.

Diseases That Dogs Can Transmit to People (Zoonotic Diseases)

Although most canine diseases are what are called "species specific"—that is, confined only to dogs—there are some canine diseases that can be transmitted to people; rabies, covered above, is the most dangerous. Generally speaking, the best protection against contagion is preventive immunization or treatment of an infected dog, when called for.

The other important step owners can take to prevent contagion is to pay strict attention to hygiene. Children in particular should be taught to automatically wash their hands after any contact with a dog or his waste and before eating, particularly if they have been playing in an area where dogs may deposit waste. Family dogs, especially those that share a bed or bedroom with a person, should be kept scrupulously clean and free from external or internal parasites. Dog runs and kennels should also be kept scrupulously clean and free of waste. Immunocompromised pet owners need to be especially careful to avoid opportunistic zoonotic infections and should discuss ways to prevent transmission with both their veterinarians and personal doctors.

Some of the most common zoonotic diseases and disorders associated with dogs are:

DOG BITES

Even if a dog is not ill, any dog bite that breaks the skin should be treated with antibiotic ointment to prevent infection. Children, especially, are often bitten on their arms or hands when playing with an overeager or overexcited puppy or dog. If redness and/or pain develop at the site of a dog bite, a doctor should be consulted so that proper antibiotics can be given if deemed necessary.

LEPTOSPIROSIS

This rather rare contagious *bacterial* disease can lead to kidney and liver disease in dogs, but rarely is transmitted to people. It is a waterborne disease, and dogs are usually infected via the urine of another infected animal. Carriers can include most farm animals and rats as well as other dogs. Humans may contract leptospirosis from the urine of an infected dog, from ingesting soil that has been urine soaked, or by drinking contaminated water. If a dog is known to have the disease, care to avoid contamination must be taken when handling him.

Signs of the disease in dogs include vomiting, loss of appetite, fever, depression, jaundice, and painful muscles. Diagnosis is made by laboratory tests, observation of symptoms, and history. Treatment consists of various antibiotics, and its success rests on early detection

and prompt attention. There is a vaccine to prevent leptospirosis in dogs, which is given selectively according to the geographic area in which a dog lives and the incidence of the disease, but may not be very effective or provide long-term immunity. A local veterinarian is the best judge of whether or not the vaccinations are needed.

RINGWORM

Ringworm is a *fungal* skin disease to which both dogs and humans, especially children, are highly susceptible. Children should not be allowed to touch a dog suspected of having the disease. It is primarily spread by direct contact, but spores can be airborne.

An affected dog will have characteristic round, hairless, scaly patches on his skin. Diagnosis is made by a veterinarian with an ultraviolet light and fungal culture. Treatment can be with topical ointment for mild cases, or with an oral medication such as griseofulvin.

PARASITES

Any parasite, such as fleas and ticks, can and will go from dogs to humans given the opportunity, carrying with them diseases such as ehrlichiosis, Lyme disease, and Rocky Mountain spotted fever. To prevent this from occurring it is important to treat an affected dog and his environment promptly. See Chapter 2, page 26, for more about this.

As we stated in Chapter 2 (page 16), roundworms (toxocara) can rarely infect people (usually children). To prevent this, dogs should be checked for worms, puppies should be wormed early, dog stools should be picked up and disposed of while fresh, and children should be taught good hygenic practices.

Care of an Injured or Sick Dog

When a pet dog is injured, an owner often must make some immediate decisions about what to do and how to do it. If a dog is ill or recuperating from surgery or injury, the owner must be prepared to look after her and tend to her needs, which may include giving medications and caring for bandages. In the case of a chronic illness such as diabetes mellitus or other long-term problems, an owner may be called on to medicate a dog for the rest of the animal's life. In this chapter we will include a brief rundown of some of the more commonly occurring emergency and recuperation situations and how to deal with them.

Emergency First Aid Steps

Most injuries and serious illnesses require immediate veterinary care, as we pointed out in Chapter 4. It is a waste of precious time for an owner to attempt first aid steps that may do more harm than good in the end. However, there are certainly situations in which something must be done to make a dog more comfortable and, perhaps, to save her life, especially in the case of traumatic injury. An owner must stop serious bleeding, try to resuscitate a dog that has drowned, and an injured dog must be transported to the veterinary office or emergency clinic in a way that will do her no further harm.

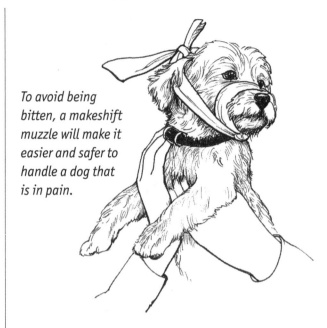

To avoid being bitten, a makeshift muzzle will make it easier and safer to handle a dog that is in pain.

A TEMPORARY MUZZLE

Common sense dictates that a dog that has serious injuries is in severe pain and is also frightened. A dog in this condition may strike out at anyone, even her owner, when she is approached

Signs of Pain

Dogs handle pain with varying degrees of stoicism, just as humans do. One dog with a slight swelling may scream as if she is in agony, while another with severe abdominal pain may act as if there is no pain.

In general, a dog in slight pain after surgery, for instance, will probably want to be left alone to rest. She will welcome a kind word or two and a gentle pat, but will not appreciate handling and may reject food for about twenty-four hours. If her discomfort lasts longer than a day, the veterinarian should be consulted.

A dog with abdominal pain sometimes adopts a posture similar to a "play bow" (see "Canine Communications," page 34), with her rear end up in the air, front legs and head down.

A dog that hurts badly will have trouble moving, may whine, groan, or cry out in pain, may pant rapidly, and possibly collapse. She may try to hide, may have trouble finding a comfortable position to lie down, and will usually completely lose her appetite. She may ask for reassurance from her owner, but will often not want to be touched and may growl, snarl, snap, or even bite if handled. An owner must take his cue from his pet as to the type and amount of attention he gives a seriously hurting dog.

Severe pain due to injury or a medical emergency is almost always accompanied by shock—see Box, page 53. Any dog that appears to have severe pain should be assessed by a veterinarian as soon as possible.

or touched. Anyone attempting to minister to an injured dog should protect his arms and hands as well as possible, and should avoid putting his face near the dog's.

If a dog is so panicky that she continuously tries to bite anyone who comes close, she may need to be temporarily muzzled. Any long strip of soft material such as a stocking, necktie, soft piece of rope, or strip of gauze will do. It is difficult for one person to apply a muzzle successfully; a helper is needed. One person should hold the dog securely from behind while the other wraps the cloth firmly around the dog's nose, crosses the ends underneath her chin, and brings them up behind her ears, where they are tied tightly. A muzzle needs to be tight or the dog will still be able to bite. A dog will still be able to breathe through her nose. See illustration, left.

TRANSPORTING AN INJURED DOG

When a dog has suffered from a traumatic injury such as a fall or being hit by a moving vehicle, it is very important to move her as little as possible to prevent further injury. But it stands to reason that if the dog is lying on a road, for instance, she must be moved quickly. It will also

be necessary to move the dog into a car or carrier to get her to a veterinarian.

A small dog can be moved one of two ways. She can be picked up with hands under her chest just behind her front legs, using two hands for support, and carried, legs dangling. This is an especially good method if a leg or legs are injured. Another way to transport a small dog is to place her in a carton or box (see illustration below).

A large, heavy dog presents more of a problem. If an owner is alone he may need to ask for help to avoid exacerbating the dog's injuries by

A small injured dog can be carried in a cardboard box.

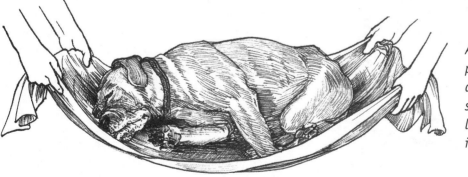

A blanket or poncho can serve as a makeshift stretcher for a large dog that is injured.

dragging her or trying to lift her by himself. Anything that can be used as a makeshift stretcher can be used to transport a large dog— a board or plank if available, or a blanket or coat held tautly by two people (see illustration, page 67).

A further caution: Even a badly injured dog may be so frightened she will try to run away. It is best if the owner can stay with an injured dog and reassure her while somebody else goes to call for help. Because of shock (see Box, page 53), it is very important to keep an injured dog as quiet as possible while help is being sought and while she is being transported.

STOPPING BLEEDING

We discussed the use of a *pressure bandage*, and how to apply one, in Chapter 4 (see page

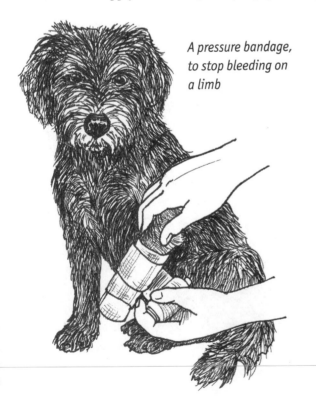

A pressure bandage, to stop bleeding on a limb

54). In the case of spurting, arterial bleeding it may be necessary to apply manual pressure with a clean cloth or bandage placed next to the wound to stop the flow of blood; then a pressure bandage can be applied. As we stated in Chapter 4, we do not advocate the use of tourniquets because they can easily cause permanent limb or extremity damage.

RESUSCITATION

If a dog is not breathing (apnea), or her heart is not beating (this can be ascertained by feeling the chest area for a heartbeat), immediate action must be taken to avoid brain damage. If the cause is electrocution from biting a plugged-in electric wire, be sure the wire is unplugged before touching the dog. If the dog almost drowned, it is important to try to get rid of as much water as possible before attempting resuscitation by tipping the dog, head down, to provide drainage. If she has vomited, take care to clear any vomitus from the airways and to tilt the dog's head down in case she regurgitates again. This prevents any regurgitated material from running down the dog's airways.

It is important to note here that, in a case of full-blown cardiac arrest, even the best-equipped intensive care facilities in major veterinary hospitals with expert staff have only a 4 percent rate of success in resuscitation. Therefore, the chances of an owner being able to successfully resuscitate a dog with cardiac arrest if he, for instance, is alone on a camping trip, are very slim. Most owners, however, feel they must at least try.

Artificial Respiration

The easiest way to perform artificial respiration to start a dog breathing again is by *mouth-to-nose resuscitation*. The dog's mouth should be sealed tightly closed using two hands, then the person's mouth should be placed firmly around the dog's nose. With gentle blowing into the nose for several seconds eight to ten times per minute, the dog may begin to breathe on her own. Once the dog has begun to breathe she should be taken to the veterinarian right away.

Cardiopulmonary Resuscitation (CPR)

If a dog has stopped breathing *and* her heart is not beating, she may be helped by CPR, a combination of heart massage and artificial respiration. As we pointed out above, however, this procedure is hardly ever successful.

The dog should be put on her right side on a hard surface. Her airways should be cleared by pulling out her tongue and checking inside her mouth and throat before beginning. First, mouth-to-nose resuscitation should be performed. If there is still no heartbeat, heart massage can be performed. A dog's heart is located in the chest just behind her front legs. With pressure appropriate for the dog's size, the heels of both hands should compress the dog's chest and then release it. This should be repeated rapidly, six to ten times, then mouth-to-nose resuscitation repeated. If no pulse is felt the process may be repeated, but if no positive results are seen after approximately ten minutes the process is probably in vain. The best course to take is to have someone try to obtain veterinary help while the resuscitation effort is under way.

Home Care of a Sick or Recuperating Dog

Inexperienced dog owners, in particular, are often very concerned about their ability to take care of or medicate a sick or recuperating dog. Owners are also often concerned about the time required to nurse a dog back to health. When an illness is serious or chronic and requires time-consuming or ongoing medication, as in the case of diabetes mellitus, for example, when treatments will be required for the rest of a dog's life, an owner must give very serious consideration as to his ability, and willingness, to proceed with treatment. The veterinarian should be consulted and told of all the owner's concerns so that she can help him make an informed decision as to how to proceed.

RESTRAINTS AND TRICKS

Some dogs are very calm and relaxed about accepting medication and treatment, even if the procedure is slightly unpleasant or painful, or the medicine doesn't taste good. Others resist unfamiliar ministrations as a general rule; they tend to be fearful when faced with any type of mild restraint or unknown procedure. If a dog is fearful she may run away and hide at the first sight of a bottle of medicine or tube of ointment. If she is truly frightened and feels threatened, she may try to bite.

With some dogs a slight distraction may help make them cooperative. A small dog is easier to handle when she is lifted up onto a counter or tabletop. A favorite treat held in one hand while the medicine is given with the other may do the trick. Sometimes a gentle tug on the ear flap will distract a dog sufficiently so she takes her medication. But a truly stubborn or fearful dog will often need to be restrained in some way before being medicated. Often a helper is needed in order to properly restrain a dog.

As we mentioned earlier in this chapter (see page 66), a homemade *muzzle* is the best protection against a dog that tries to bite because of fear or pain.

Another way to restrain a large dog is with *manual restraint*. A helper can place the animal's head firmly underneath his armpit and hold it there while the dog is medicated. Or, a dog can be held tightly against a helper's body with two arms, one around the neck, the other underneath the dog's stomach in front of the hind legs.

If a dog immediately tries to lick off any ointment or salve, or chew off a bandage, it may

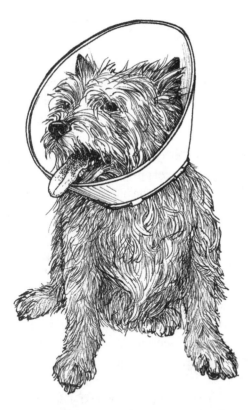

An Elizabethan collar will prevent a dog from scratching her head or ears, licking ointment or salve off her body, or chewing a bandage. The collar must be removed at intervals, under strict supervision, to allow the dog to eat and drink.

be necessary to use an *Elizabethan collar* (see illustration below). This is a soft plastic cone, available from a veterinarian, that ties around the animal's neck behind her ears and extends beyond the tip of her nose so that she cannot get her mouth to any part of her body or scratch any part of her head or ears. Most dogs really hate these devices, but they are sometimes necessary on a temporary basis. The collar must be removed at intervals, under supervision, to allow a dog to eat and drink.

GENERAL DAILY CARE OF A SICK DOG

A dog that is sick or recuperating from an operation or accident is in a somewhat fragile condition—that is, she is apt to be more sensitive to extremes of temperature—and more bothered by loud noise and commotion. Just as with a human patient, a dog that doesn't feel well should be kept warm and protected from rough-housing children. Even sick dogs, however, usually do not want to be completely isolated from their families, so every effort should be made to find a warm, quiet corner somewhere where the patient can still see and hear normal household activities. A dog's own bed may be the ideal spot when she is recovering, as long as it is in a draft-free, traffic-free location. An extra blanket or quilt may make her more comfortable. Sometimes a dog is too sick to go outdoors or her illness may cause her to have diarrhea. If this is the case, a plastic sheet placed underneath a washable blanket or towel will help; the bedding on top must be changed frequently to be sure it is kept clean.

An owner may be asked by the veterinarian to *take the dog's temperature* on a regular basis. The veterinarian should demonstrate how to do this, but basically the temperature is taken with a standard rectal thermometer, lubricated with Vaseline. After the thermometer is shaken down it is placed gently into the dog's rectum until only one inch remains visible. It should remain in place for one minute. A normal temperature for a dog is between 100 and 102.5 degrees. If it is above that, the dog has a fever; if it is below, the dog is hypothermic and needs to be kept warmer. Again, placing a small dog on a counter or table-top will make this process easier.

If a dog is very ill she may have trouble getting up to eat or drink regularly, so her food and water bowls should be placed within easy reach. If she is refusing to eat and drink altogether, she may have to be *forcefed,* at least for a while. To force fluids, use a large dropper or syringe, available from a veterinarian or pharmacist. Place the fluid in the dropper or syringe and, with the dog's head tilted upward, pull her cheek out gently using a thumb and finger (see illustration below). Slowly allow the fluid to gather in the funnel-like opening created by the cheek pouch so it can flow into the animal's mouth through her teeth. To give solid nourishment, put some strained baby food or prescription food from a veterinarian in a syringe and squeeze it into the dog's mouth. Alternately, use a tongue depressor and wipe the food on the roof of the dog's mouth behind the top front teeth.

MEDICATING A DOG

If an owner has not had any experience medicating a dog, he should not hesitate to ask the veterinarian for detailed instructions and a demonstration as to how to best give whatever medication is required. Dogs differ greatly in their willingness to take medication, as they do with all other medical procedures.

Liquid medicine is probably the easiest to give, following the instructions for forcefeeding liquids, above.

Pills and capsules that are flavored usually present no problems at all. If they are not flavored and a dog has retained her appetite, they can be hidden inside a ball of meat, bread, or cheese and

Liquid nutrients or medication can be placed in a large syringe and squeezed into a dog's mouth.

Pilling a dog. Note where the pill should be placed.

fed to the dog. This works well for most dogs, but some will eat the meat, bread, or cheese and spit out the pill or capsule. If a dog is not eating well, or spits out a disguised capsule or pill, the medicine will have to be given by hand. If the capsule is large, it helps to grease it with a little oil or butter. Grasping the dog's muzzle from the top with one hand, tilt her head up. Force the lower part of her jaw open and toss the pill into the back of her throat, then push it gently into her throat with a finger (see illustration, page 71). Hold the dog's mouth closed with one hand and massage her throat downward to force her to swallow. Be sure she actually does swallow or the entire procedure will have to be repeated. Caution: Do *not* put medicine in a dog's dinner. She

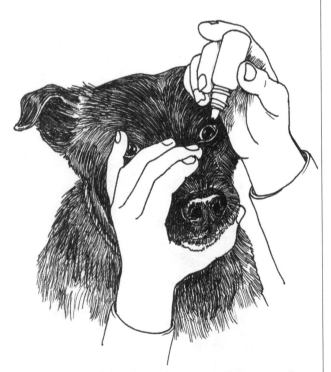

When applying drops, be very careful not to poke the dog in the eye. Rest your hand on top of the animal's head to steady it.

may not eat all of her food, or she might eat it all and go somewhere and spit out the pill.

Eye medicine comes in two forms, liquid drops or ointment. Whichever form it is in, it is important to be extremely careful not to poke the dog's eye when applying it. Hold the dog firmly underneath her chin and tilt her head upward. Rest the other hand on top of the dog's head to steady it and place the tip of the applicator at the inner edge of her eye next to the nose (see illustration below). Squeeze the medicine directly into the dog's eye, then close the lid over the medicine to help spread it over the eye.

To give *ear medicine,* either liquid or ointment, hold the dog's ear flap and place the tip of the applicator vertically into the dog's ear canal opening and squeeze. Still holding the ear flap, gently remove the applicator while still squeezing so the ointment coats the entire ear canal. Continue to hold the dog's ear and gently massage the area right beneath the ear to spread the medicine. It is usually possible to feel a dog's ear canal on the side of her head. Continue to massage for as long as possible.

Skin ointments and salves are generally fairly easy to apply. Problems can occur, however, if a dog immediately begins to lick them off. Sometimes a distraction such as a treat, game of fetch, or short walk on a leash will prevent a dog from licking the medicine off for as long as it takes (approximately ten minutes) to penetrate the skin and begin to work. If a dog cannot be distracted from licking medication off her skin, however, it may be necessary to use an Elizabethan collar (see page 70), especially at night when no one is watching the dog.

If a dog requires *injections* at home, the veterinarian will demonstrate how to give them.

Sometimes *medicated baths* are prescribed,

especially for skin conditions. Follow the instructions for "Bathing a Dog" in Chapter 2, page 25.

Casts and Bandages

Casts and bandages are usually left alone between veterinary visits. The hardest job for an owner is to keep them dry and as clean as possible. A heavy plastic trash bag cut in pieces and attached with adhesive or masking tape is usually somewhat effective in protecting a cast or bandage from snow, rain, or mud when a dog is outdoors. (Note: Do *not* apply tape to fur or it will be impossible to get off without pulling the fur. Instead, attach the tape to the plastic bag itself.) The plastic must be taken off as soon as the dog comes indoors to prevent dampness and bacteria from building up underneath it.

If a dog persistently chews on a bandage or cast, or continuously licks the area around it, it may be necessary to use an Elizabethan collar (see page 70) to prevent soreness and infection from developing. If an owner notices any swelling or irritation around a cast or bandage or in any part of a bandaged limb, such as a foot if the leg is bandaged, the veterinarian should be contacted immediately. One of the most dangerous situations involving casts and bandages occurs when the bandage slips down the leg or when the bandage is too tight. In either case, circulation to the foot and toes may be cut off, causing the foot and toes to swell. A properly applied leg bandage should leave toes exposed at the bottom. The owner must check the toes by sight and feel several times a day. If any swelling occurs, the dog should be seen by a veterinarian as soon as possible.

Part Three

More Than 180

of the Most Commonly Seen

Canine Signs / Symptoms

of Illness and

How to Interpret Them

Index of
More Than
180 Signs/
Symptoms *

*Bold entries are alphabetically listed as headings in "More Than 180 of the Most Commonly Seen Canine Signs/Symptoms of Illness and How to Interpret Them," pp. 89–153.

Anorexia (Appetite Loss)—see
> **Abdominal Distension;**
> **Appetite, Abnormal;**
> **Depression/Lethargy;**
> **Diarrhea;**
> **Ear Problems;**
> **Eye Disorders;**
> **Mouth Disorders;**
> **Mucous Membrane Color;**
> **Thirst, Changes in;**
> **Urination, Abnormal;**
> **Vomiting;**
> see also "Signs of Pain," Box, p. 66;
> "Pyometra," pp. 51 and 113

Appetite, Abnormal—see also
> **Diarrhea;**
> **Thirst, Changes in;**
> "Eating Behavior," p. 30

Aural Hematoma—see
> **Ear Problems**

Bad Breath—see
> **Mouth Disorders;**
> **Thirst, Changes in**

Balance Loss—see
> **Ear Problems;**
> **Incoordination;**
> see also Appendix A: Some Common
> Household Products That Are Poisonous,
> pp. 157–58

Barking, inappropriate—see
> **Abnormal Geriatric Behavior;**
> **Ear Problems;**
> see also p. 38

Begging for Food—see
> **Appetite, Abnormal**

Behavior, Abnormal—see
> **Abnormal Geriatric Behavior;**
> **Depression/Lethargy;**
> **Incoordination;**
> see also pp. 36–38; "Rabies," p. 59; "Signs
> of Pain," p. 66; Appendix A: Some
> Common Household Products That Are
> Poisonous, pp. 157–58

Biting—see
> "Canine Communications," pp. 31–35;
> "Aggressive Behavior," pp. 36–37; "Signs of
> Pain," Box, p. 66

Bleeding—see
> **Nasal Disorders;**
> see also pp. 48–49, 53–54

Blindness—see
> **Eye Disorders;**
> **Depression/Lethargy;**
> see also Appendix A: Some Common
> Household Products That Are Poisonous,
> pp. 157–58

Bloating—see
> **Abdominal Distension**

Blood in Stool—see
> **Diarrhea;**
> see also Appendix A: Some Common
> Household Products That Are Poisonous,
> pp. 157–58

Retained Baby Teeth—see
Mouth Disorders

Salivation, excessive—see
Abdominal Distension;
Gagging;
see also Appendix A: Some Common
Household Products That Are Poisonous,
pp. 157–58

Scabs—see
Nasal Disorders;
Ear Problems

Scooting Rear End on Floor—see
Rectal Problems

Scratching—see
Ear Problems;
Eye Disorders;
Skin Disorders

Seizures—see
Depression/Lethargy;
Incoordination;
see also "Hypoglycemia," p. 51;
"Seizures/Convulsions," pp. 51–52;
"Cryptococcosis," p. 60; Appendix A: Some
Common Household Products That Are
Poisonous, pp. 157–58

Skin Disorders—see also
"Blastomycosis," p. 60; "Ringworm," p. 63

Skin, thin—see
Abdominal Distension

Skin, yellow—see
Mucous Membrane Color

Snapping—see
"Signs of Pain," Box, p. 66

Snarling—see
"Dominance Aggression," p. 32; "Signs of
Pain," Box, p. 66

Sneezing—see
Gagging;
Nasal Disorders;
Respiratory Difficulties

Snoring—see
Nasal Disorders;
Respiratory Difficulties

Snorting—see
Gagging;
Nasal Disorders;
see also "Reverse Sneezing," Box, p. 139

Spinal Problems/Disorders—see
Depression/Lethargy;
Incoordination;
Lameness

Spitting Out Food—see
Appetite, Abnormal;
Mouth Disorders

Squinting—see
Eye Disorders

Stair Difficulty—see
Lameness;
see also "Signs of Pain," Box, p. 66

Stealing Food—see
Appetite, Abnormal

More Than 180 of the Most Commonly Seen Canine Signs/Symptoms of Illness and How to Interpret Them

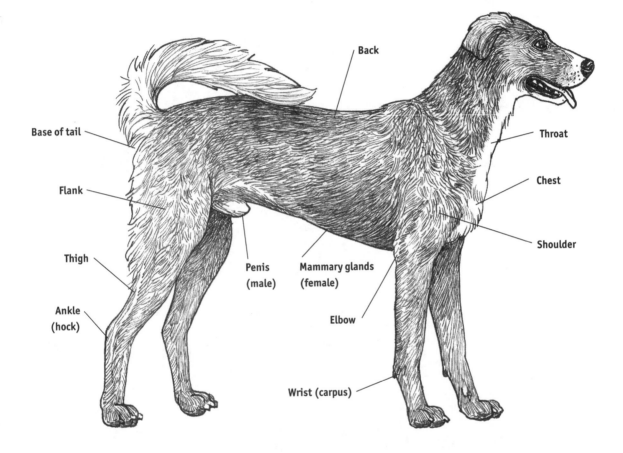

Side View of a Dog

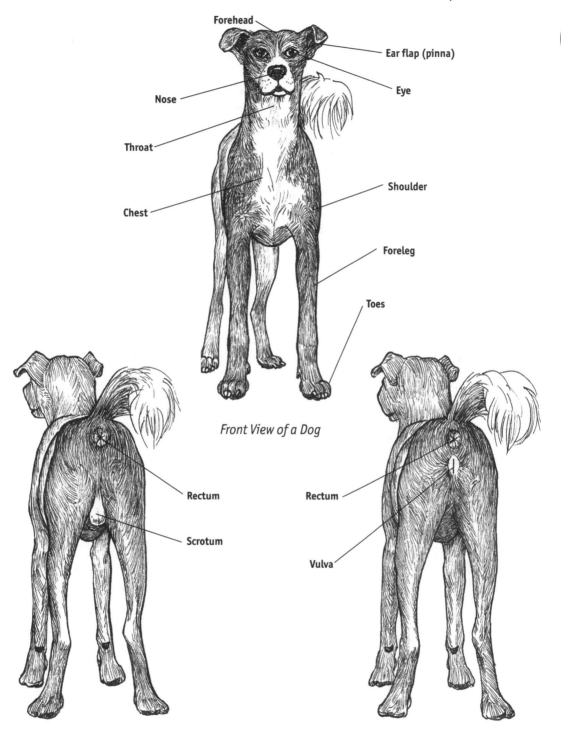

Forehead

Ear flap (pinna)

Eye

Nose

Throat

Shoulder

Chest

Foreleg

Toes

Front View of a Dog

Rectum

Scrotum

Rectum

Vulva

Rear View of an Unneutered Male Dog

Rear View of a Female Dog

Abdominal Distension

Any change in the outward shape or size of a dog's abdomen should be carefully assessed. A dog's abdomen may appear larger than normal due to pregnancy, excess fat accumulation either in the abdomen itself or underneath the surrounding skin, a buildup of gas or fluid in the stomach or intestines, an infection that causes swelling, an obstruction in the urinary tract, a growth or enlargement of an internal organ.

Sign/Symptom	Observations	Associated Signs	Possible Condition	Action to Take
Chronic abdominal distension	Dog feels fine	None	Obesity	✚ Low-calorie diet. Reduce number of treats. 📞 See veterinarian for guidelines
Chronic abdominal distension	Dog feels fine	Panting. Increased thirst. Increased urination. Hair loss. Thin skin.	Cushing's syndrome (see Glossary for definition)	📞 See veterinarian for endocrine testing
Intact female dog. Progressive abdominal distension.	Dog feels fine. Was in heat approximately two months ago.	Increased appetite. Milk in mammary glands (see also Mammary Gland Abnormalities).	Pregnancy	📞 See veterinarian for diagnosis
Intact female dog. Progressive abdominal distension.	Vaginal discharge and lethargy	Increased thirst and urination. Possible vomiting, decreased appetite.	Pyometra (uterine infection). See Box, p. 113; see also p. 51.	⊕ See veterinarian for X ray, blood tests, surgery

✚ Home care; first aid   📞 Call veterinarian   📞24 Call veterinarian; make appointment within 24 hours

Sign/Symptom	Observations	Associated Signs	Possible Condition	Action to Take
Progressive abdominal distension, acute or chronic	Dog may be weak, losing weight, acting lethargic	Weight loss. Muscle loss. Vomiting. Decreased appetite. Diarrhea.	Abdominal mass. Enlarged liver or spleen. Cancer. Peritonitis (see Glossary). Ascites (see Glossary) from liver or heart failure.	See veterinarian for X rays and other tests, possible surgery
Progressive, acute abdominal distension	Dog is not urinating and/or straining to urinate	Anorexia and/or vomiting. Lethargy.	Obstructed urinary tract	Go to emergency clinic for X rays, tests, surgery
Acute abdominal distension	Weakness and/or collapse	Pale mucous membranes	Hemorrhage into abdominal cavity due to ingestion of rodenticide. Ruptured spleen or tumor. Cancer. Abdominal hematoma.	Go to emergency clinic for X rays, tests, surgery
Acute abdominal distension	Restlessness. Retching. Salivating. Trembling. Usually large, deep-chested dog.	Collapse. Painful abdomen. Pale mucous membranes.	GDV—gastric dilatation/volvulus ("Bloat"). See pp. 50–51.	Go to emergency clinic for shock treatment, gastric decompression, surgery

Call veterinarian; make appointment immediately   Life-threatening condition; go *immediately* to veterinarian or emergency clinic

Abnormal Geriatric Behavior

This is technically called *cognitive dysfunction,* or the canine equivalent of Alzheimer's disease. It includes a variety of behavior changes that indicate the dog has lost touch with previously learned traits and patterns. Until recently, this was essentially untreatable, and often led eventually to situations in which the dog could no longer be kept as a pet. Now, approximately 75 percent of dogs with this condition respond at least partially to medical therapy.

Sign/Symptom	Observations	Associated Signs	Possible Condition	Action to Take
Abnormal behavior in an old dog	Disorientation: becoming trapped in unusual locations; inappropriate nocturnal barking; loss of housebreaking; sleeping during the day and pacing at night; not recognizing familiar people	Anything associated with old age (e.g., blindness, deafness, arthritis)	Cognitive dysfunction. Serious liver disease. Brain disease, including tumor.	See veterinarian. Medical therapy (L-Deprenyl) available for cognitive disorders. Workup needed to rule out other conditions.

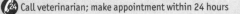
Home care; first aid   Call veterinarian   Call veterinarian; make appointment within 24 hours

Appetite, Abnormal

Dogs' normal appetites vary greatly, from voracious to picky. It becomes a concern when a dog's eating habits change suddenly. There are three distinct types of appetite a dog may exhibit that can be called "abnormal": a *decrease* in a dog's normal appetite; an *increase* in a dog's normal appetite; and the eating of *inappropriate things* (pica or coprophagia). A dog that stops eating entirely can usually survive for many days as long as she drinks water daily.

Sign/Symptom	Observations	Associated Signs	Possible Condition	Action to Take
Increase in appetite	Begging for food; stealing food	Increase in weight. Normal bowels.	Feeding more palatable diet. Behavioral.	Decrease amount fed if weight gain or feed a low-calorie diet. Consult veterinarian or behaviorist for possible behavioral cause.
Sudden increase in appetite	Begging for food; stealing food	Drinking a lot more water. Distended abdomen. Hair loss.	Cushing's disease (see Glossary)	Call veterinarian for laboratory tests
Sudden increase in appetite	Begging for food; stealing food	Drinking a lot more water. Weight loss.	Diabetes mellitus (see Glossary)	(24) Consult veterinarian for laboratory tests
Ravenous appetite (often young German shepherds)	Eats food rapidly in great quantities	Weight loss. Thin, poor haircoat. Often voluminous, soft, foul-smelling stools.	EPI—exocrine pancreatic insufficiency (see Glossary)	Consult veterinarian for laboratory tests. Can be treated with diet therapy and medication.
Decreased appetite	Acts normal. No vomiting or diarrhea.	None	Aversion to food given. Prefers "people food."	Feed normal diet, and be patient. If weight loss, consult veterinarian

Call veterinarian; make appointment immediately

Life-threatening condition; go *immediately* to veterinarian or emergency clinic

Sign/Symptom	Observations	Associated Signs	Possible Condition	Action to Take
Decreased appetite	May spit out food	Drooling, possibly bloody saliva. Paws at mouth.	Bad tooth. Oral lesion or tumor. Foreign body caught on tooth or across roof of mouth. Mouth infection.	➕ Examine mouth for stick/bone caught across roof of mouth 🕔 Have veterinarian assess dental status. If unusual mass or masses are noted, consult veterinarian.
Decreased appetite	Not feeling well. Acting quiet.	Drooling; vomiting; burping	Nausea—see Vomiting	See Vomiting
Decreased appetite	Lethargic	None	Nonspecific fever	➕ Take temperature (see pp. 70–71) 🕔 If temperature is 102.5–104.5, consult veterinarian ⊕ If temperature is greater than 104.5, seek immediate veterinary help
Eats unnatural things such as dirt, stones, cat litter (pica)	Often young, active dog	Sometimes constipated from foreign material	Behavioral. Stress. Genetic predisposition.	➕ Try to eliminate stress. Eliminate access to specific foreign material. 📞 Consult veterinarian and/or behaviorist

➕ Home care; first aid   📞 Call veterinarian   🕔 Call veterinarian; make appointment within 24 hours

Sign/Symptom	Observations	Associated Signs	Possible Condition	Action to Take
Eats stools (coprophagia)	Usually eats own stool, occasionally other dogs'. (Many dogs will eat cat stools if given the opportunity.)	None	Any case of increased appetite (see above), or intestinal disease (see Diarrhea). Possible genetic predisposition.	✚ Try meat tenderizer or pancreatic enzymes in food. Commercial products (FORBID) may be added to food to impart a bad taste to stools. ✆ Take to veterinarian for tests to determine if there is a medical problem

A

P
P
E
T
I
T
E
,

A
B
N
O
R
M
A
L

 Call veterinarian; make appointment immediately   Life-threatening condition; go *immediately* to veterinarian or emergency clinic

Depression/Lethargy

A dog is considered *depressed* if he exhibits general malaise, is obviously ill, and shows no interest in his surroundings. If he is depressed, a dog that normally loves to play fetch, for instance, will not get up when a ball is tossed. He may lose interest in food and may not even respond to loving attention. At the same time he may be *lethargic*. That is, he will be quieter than usual and, again, disinterested in what's going on around him. These conditions always signal pain and/or some type of systemic disease or disorder. A dog that is suffering from depression and/or lethargy should be evaluated by a veterinarian as soon as possible.

Sign/Symptom	Observations	Associated Signs	Possible Condition	Action to Take
Depression/lethargy	Coughing. Rapid breathing. Difficulty breathing.	Anorexia and weight loss	Heart failure (see "Cardiovascular Emergencies," pp. 49–50). Pneumonia. Pleural (lung) fluid. Lung cancer.	Go to emergency clinic for a chest X ray
Depression/lethargy	Lameness. Weakness or paralysis.	Obvious pain. Reluctance to walk.	Muscle disease. Arthritis (degenerative; immune; infectious—see Glossary). Bone tumor. Spinal disease. Intervertebral disc disease.	See veterinarian for X rays, blood tests, medication

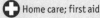 Home care; first aid   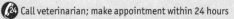 Call veterinarian   Call veterinarian; make appointment within 24 hours

Sign/Symptom	Observations	Associated Signs	Possible Condition	Action to Take
Depression/lethargy	Increased thirst and urination	Anorexia. Vomiting. Weight loss.	Kidney failure. Kidney infection. Liver disease. Pyometra (uterine infection—see p. 51; see also Box, p. 113). Diabetes mellitus (see Glossary).	Go to emergency clinic for blood tests, urinalysis, cultures, and possible surgery
Depression/lethargy	Vomiting. Diarrhea.	Anorexia. Weight loss.	Enteritis (bacterial or viral—see Glossary). Foreign body in the gastrointestinal tract. Cancer of the gastrointestinal tract. Pancreatitis (inflammation of the pancreas).	Bring fecal sample to the veterinarian, who will also perform X rays and blood tests
Depression/lethargy	Rectal temperature over 103 degrees F. (see pp. 70–71)	Anorexia	Infection of the: organs (e.g., kidneys); blood system; joints; body cavities. External abscess.	Go to emergency clinic for tests and/or X rays
Depression/lethargy	Dog seems to be in pain	Reluctance to move. Cries when touched.	Polyarthropathy (joint disease throughout the body). Muscle inflammation. Neck or back pain. Abdominal pain.	Go to emergency clinic for X rays, joint taps, etc.

D

E P R E S S I O N / L E T H A R G Y

 Call veterinarian; make appointment immediately   Life-threatening condition; go *immediately* to veterinarian or emergency clinic

Sign/Symptom	Observations	Associated Signs	Possible Condition	Action to Take
Depression/lethargy	Weakness. Collapse.	Pale mucous membranes	Anemia, caused by: blood loss; red blood cell destruction (hemolytic anemia); bone marrow disease (aplastic anemia)—see Glossary. Shock caused by trauma, fluid loss, blood loss, bacterial infection.	⊕ Go to emergency clinic for blood tests and treatment
Depression/lethargy	Weakness. Collapse.	Improves when dog eats	Low blood sugar, due to: liver disease; insulin secreting tumor; for small, young dog, see "Hypoglycemia," p. 51.	✆ Feed frequently. See veterinarian for blood tests. ⊕ If collapse, give oral sugar (see p. 51)
Depression/lethargy	Dementia. Blindness. Stupor. Coma. Seizures. Behavior changes.	Signs become worse after dog eats (if liver failure)	Liver failure. Brain tumor. Inflammatory nervous system disease (e.g., encephalitis). Drugs/toxins in system.	⊕ Withhold food ⊕ Go to emergency clinic
Depression/lethargy	Overweight. Thin haircoat. Dandruff.	Prefers warm places	Hypothyroidism	✆ See veterinarian for endocrine testing

⊕ Home care; first aid   ✆ Call veterinarian   ✆24 Call veterinarian; make appointment within 24 hours

D

Diarrhea

Diarrhea is fairly common in dogs and is often due to their tendency to eat spoiled food, garbage, and whatever else they can find. It can be caused by other dietary factors as well, such as eating table scraps or treats that are too rich, a change in diet, or too much food. Chronic diarrhea is usually accompanied by weight loss or, in the case of puppies, failure to gain appropriately. It can be caused by a roundworm infestation (see page 16) or a digestive tract disorder. If diarrhea is limited to one or two sudden attacks and the dog appears to be lively and continues to have an appetite, an owner can afford a "wait and see" approach. If, however, the diarrhea lasts for more than twenty-four hours, a dog is also vomiting, is in obvious distress, there is blood in the stool, or the dog becomes lethargic, it can indicate a serious or life-threatening condition such as canine distemper (see page 58), parvovirus (see pages 58–59), or hemorrhagic gastroenteritis (HGE), a serious intestinal disease (see Box, below). See Box, page 105, "Home Treatment of Routine Diarrhea or Vomiting."

Hemorrhagic Gastroenteritis (HGE)

This is a noncontagious disease that has no known cause. It occurs suddenly, and small dogs are particularly apt to develop HGE, especially miniature dachshunds, miniature schnauzers, and toy poodles. It is marked by a large volume of bloody, foul-smelling diarrhea that may be accompanied by vomiting. This is a severe, life-threatening emergency. A dog with HGE must be given intravenous fluids immediately, accompanied by antibiotics. A dog with untreated HGE will quickly collapse, go into shock (see Box, page 53), and die.

Call veterinarian; make appointment immediately

 Life-threatening condition; go *immediately* to veterinarian or emergency clinic

Sign/Symptom	Observations	Associated Signs	Possible Condition	Action to Take
Acute, one to several times	Watery; yellow to brown	None	Dietary indiscretion; simple enteritis (see Glossary); overeating; diet change; intestinal parasites; viral infection; bacterial infection	✚ Treat for routine diarrhea 📞 If continues, see the veterinarian for examination, medication; bring fecal sample
Acute, one to several times	Doesn't respond to home treatment (see Box, p. 105)	Possible dehydration (see p. 152); possible lethargy; possible anorexia	Viral infection; bacterial infection; intestinal parasites; food poisoning; Addison's disease (see Glossary); reaction to antibiotic therapy; inflammatory bowel disease (IBD—see Glossary)	📞24 See the veterinarian for examination, tests, medication
Acute, one to several times	Anorexia; lethargy; depression; dehydration (see p. 152)	Possible fever; possible weakness; possible vomiting	Viral infection, such as parvovirus (pp. 58–59) or distemper (p. 58). Bacterial infection. IBD (see Glossary). Addison's disease (see Glossary). Food poisoning. Intestinal parasites. Kidney disease. Liver disease. Peritonitis (see Glossary). Partial obstruction.	📞24 See the veterinarian for examination, tests, medication

✚ Home care; first aid   📞 Call veterinarian   📞24 Call veterinarian; make appointment within 24 hours

Sign/Symptom	Observations	Associated Signs	Possible Condition	Action to Take
Acute, one to several times	Flecks, streaks, or clots of bright red blood in stool and/or mucus in stool	Straining to defecate. Frequent defecation.	Colitis (see Glossary). Hookworms. Whipworms. Giardia. Rectal/colon tumor. Bone chips in rectum.	See the veterinarian for treatment. Take stool sample.
Acute, one to several times	Defecates large pools of bright or dark blood	Vomiting	HGE (see Box, p. 101). Parvovirus (see pp. 58–59). Bleeding disorder. Addison's disease (see Glossary).	Go to the emergency clinic for fluids, medication
Acute, one to several times	Long, white coiled worms passed in stool	Vomiting	Roundworms	See the veterinarian for medication. Take stool sample.
Passes small pieces of white material in the stool that look like rice	Healthy dog. May "scoot" on floor.	Dog has fleas, or has had fleas	Tapeworms	See the veterinarian for medication. Take stool sample.
Chronic diarrhea	No weight loss; dog acts normal	None	Food allergy or diet intolerance	Change diet / Call veterinarian for advice
Chronic diarrhea	No weight loss; dog acts normal	Possible vomiting	Parasites. Inflammatory bowel disease (IBD—see Glossary). Bacterial infection.	See the veterinarian for medication, possible tests. Take stool sample.
Chronic diarrhea	Increased appetite	Weight loss	Bacterial infection. Malabsorption. Exocrine pancreatic insufficiency (EPI— see Glossary).	See the veterinarian for tests. Take stool sample.

D

I
A
R
R
H
E
A

Call veterinarian; make appointment immediately   Life-threatening condition; go *immediately* to veterinarian or emergency clinic

Sign/Symptom	Observations	Associated Signs	Possible Condition	Action to Take
Chronic diarrhea	Anorexia. Dehydration (see p. 152). Depression.	Weight loss; possible vomiting	Viral infection. Bacterial infection. Fungal disease. Intestinal parasites. Kidney disorder. Liver disorder. Addison's disease (see Glossary). Partial intestinal obstruction. Intestinal tumor. Inflammatory bowel disease (IBD—see Glossary). Peritonitis (see Glossary).	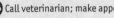 See the veterinarian for fluids, tests
Chronic diarrhea	Poor appetite; possible vomiting; weight loss	Swelling of limbs (edema)	Intestinal lymphangiectasia (dilatation of the intestinal lymphatic system)	See the veterinarian for tests, biopsy

Home care; first aid   Call veterinarian   Call veterinarian; make appointment within 24 hours

Home Treatment of Routine Diarrhea or Vomiting

If a dog is suffering from diarrhea or is vomiting and seems to be in good general health otherwise, the first thing to do is withhold all food for twenty-four hours and restrict water intake to small drinks every few hours. If a dog is vomiting a great deal, water should be restricted to *very* small amounts, or give ice cubes until she stops. (Withholding all water may lead to dehydration.) This gives the dog's digestive system a rest and prevents the loss of fluids from the body, which might cause dehydration. After the dog has stopped vomiting, give her more ice cubes. If they are kept down, somewhat larger amounts of water can then be given gradually. A mild antacid is sometimes recommended by veterinarians. After twenty-four hours, a small amount of bland food can be offered. Well-cooked white rice mixed with pieces of skinless chicken breast that has been boiled to remove any fat (three parts rice to one part chicken) is usually well tolerated and binding. This diet should be given for several days after a bout of diarrhea or vomiting. If the vomiting or diarrhea persists, further veterinary evaluation is needed. *Warning:* Withholding food for twenty-four hours in very small dogs or puppies may lead to hypoglycemia (low blood sugar) and is dangerous. In this instance, withhold food for several hours and administer small amounts of honey, Karo syrup, or sugar water (see page 51) frequently during the period of food withdrawal.

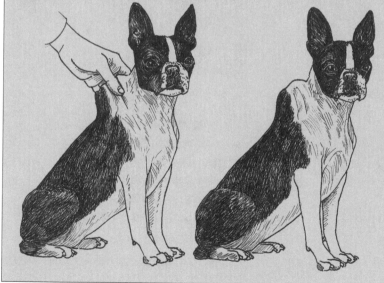

When a dog is dehydrated, her skin will lose its elasticity and will not bounce back immediately when grasped, but will tent momentarily. Dehydration occurs when there is a decreased intake of water for whatever reason or increased water loss due to overheating, diarrhea, illness, high fever, etc.

 Call veterinarian; make appointment immediately

Life-threatening condition; go *immediately* to veterinarian or emergency clinic

Ear Problems

When a dog has an ear problem, she usually lets her owner know by either scratching her ears or shaking her head. If an owner sees a noticeable increase of either sign, he should examine the ears for redness, discharge, or unusual odor. Sometimes a dog will show pain when her ears are manipulated, but because of the anatomy of a dog's ear canal (see illustration, below), the problem may be so deep that it is not easily seen and can be diagnosed only with an otoscope. Painful inner or middle ear infections that often affect children are not commonly seen in dogs.

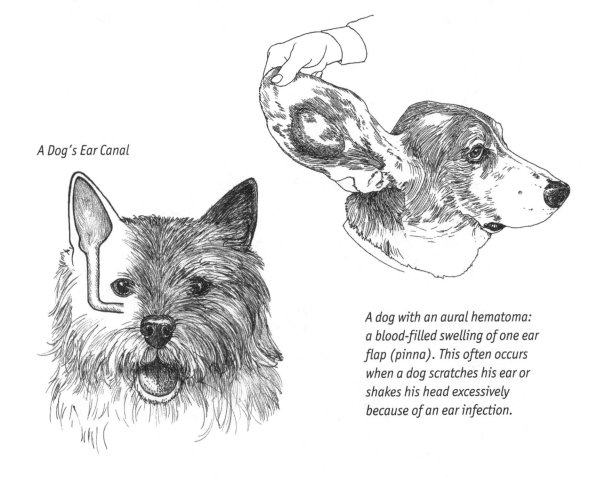

A Dog's Ear Canal

A dog with an aural hematoma: a blood-filled swelling of one ear flap (pinna). This often occurs when a dog scratches his ear or shakes his head excessively because of an ear infection.

✚ Home care; first aid   ✆ Call veterinarian   ✆₂₄ Call veterinarian; make appointment within 24 hours

Sign/Symptom	Observations	Associated Signs	Possible Condition	Action to Take
Shaking head or scratching ears	May seem unhappy	Odor from ears. Discharge inside ear—dark, orange waxy substance, or purulent (pussy) substance.	External ear infection (infection of the ear canal)	Remove hair from ear canals, if present. Clean ears with ear-cleaning solution. See veterinarian for medication.
Shaking head	Puppy or dog living with cats that go outdoors	Possible minimal dark wax in ears	Ear mites	See veterinarian for microscopic diagnosis. Treat with product designed to eradicate mites
Swelling of ear flap (pinna)	Acute onset. Feels soft. May be small, or may involve most of ear flap. Not painful.	May shake head or hold head to one side	Aural hematoma	See veterinarian to drain or operate and treat possible underlying infection
Swelling of ear flap (pinna)	Hot-feeling and painful to the touch	May shake head and hold head to one side	Infected ear flap secondary to bite wound or injury	See veterinarian for antibiotics and possible draining
Crusts and scabs along edge of ear flap	Affects erect-eared dogs in the summertime	None. Sometimes scratches ears.	Fly bites	Keep dog in house. Use insect repellents recommended by a veterinarian. Apply veterinarian-recommended antibiotic/cortisone ointment.

E
A
R

P
R
O
B
L
E
M
S

Sign/Symptom	Observations	Associated Signs	Possible Condition	Action to Take
One or both ear flaps acutely thickened	Dog may seem uncomfortable. Scratching.	May rub face, shake head	Acute allergic reaction (insect bite likely)	✚ Can give veterinarian-recommended antihistamines or oral cortisone 📞24 If continues, see veterinarian for an injection
Head tilt—also see Incoordination— canine idiopathic vestibular syndrome	May not want to walk. Appetite poor. May act nauseated or vomit.	May fall to side of head tilt. May be incoordinated. Signs of external ear infection.	Inner or middle ear infection	📞24 See veterinarian for tests, antibiotics. May require surgery.
Loss of hearing	Doesn't respond to normal sounds or commands. May seem to come on suddenly.	May bark at inappropriate times	Puppies—congenital hearing impairment (especially Dalmatians). Old dogs—geriatric hearing loss.	📞 May be evaluated at some veterinary institutions

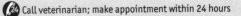

✚ Home care; first aid   📞 Call veterinarian   📞24 Call veterinarian; make appointment within 24 hours

Eye Disorders

The eye is perhaps the hardest part of a dog's body for an owner to evaluate. Many signs an owner may notice are manifestations of problems within the eye, and this is an area that cannot be properly diagnosed without special equipment. In addition, unless an owner is familiar with the correct descriptive terms, it can be difficult for her to accurately explain to the veterinarian what she has observed. If an eye looks different it probably has internal changes.

Most veterinarians are familiar with, and capable of treating, many commonly seen ocular disorders. However, there have been great advancements in treating more complicated eye problems. Very often, a veterinarian will refer an owner to a veterinary ophthalmologist, who has the expertise and equipment to deal with difficult cases.

If a dog is exhibiting any signs of an eye problem that do not match those below, it is advisable to consult a veterinarian soon.

Sign/Symptom	Observations	Associated Signs	Possible Condition	Action to Take
Mucoid discharge from one or both eyes	May come and go. Dog does not squint.	White portion of eye bloodshot. Discharge may be yellow to green.	Conjunctivitis (see Glossary), due to irritant, infection, abnormality of the lids, eyelashes	Antibiotic ophthalmic ointment recommended by the veterinarian; If unresponsive, see veterinarian for evaluation and medication
Thick, stringy discharge, one or both eyes	Usually chronic	Eventual changes in cornea	Dry eye (lack of tears)	See veterinarian for medication
Eye partially or completely out of socket	Usually occurs in brachycephalic breeds	Lethargy. Signs of pain.	Proptosed globe	Go immediately to emergency clinic. Time is critical if eye is to be saved.

Call veterinarian; make appointment immediately

Life-threatening condition; go *immediately* to veterinarian or emergency clinic

Sign/Symptom	Observations	Associated Signs	Possible Condition	Action to Take
Squinting	Seems uncomfortable	Affected eye bloodshot and tearing	Corneal ulcer. (Also possible manifestation of deeper eye problem.)	See veterinarian, who will look for underlying reason for ulcer and treat with medication, rarely surgery
Swollen eyelids	Rapid onset	Scratches face	Allergic reaction	Give antihistamines/ cortisone, as recommended by veterinarian. If not responding, see veterinarian
Pupils are unequal size	Dog may squint	Eye(s) may tear	Corneal ulcer. Inflammation inside of eye. Ocular or brain tumor. Trauma.	See veterinarian. If dog is in pain
Eye appears larger than normal/pushed forward	Appetite loss. Lethargy.	Painful if mouth is opened	Abscess or tumor behind eye	See veterinarian for assessment
Cloudy cornea (see Glossary)	Eye may look larger. If both eyes, may have visual deficit.	None	Edema (swelling) of the cornea. Possibly glaucoma (see Glossary).	Go to emergency clinic for treatment
Cloudy lens	None	Possible vision deficit	Cataracts (see Glossary). Older dog— nuclear (lenticular) sclerosis. See Box, right.	See veterinarian
Gradual vision loss	Reluctant to go out at night. Bumps into walls/objects.	Seizures. Personality changes. Other neurological signs.	Brain tumor	See veterinarian

+ Home care; first aid   Call veterinarian   Call veterinarian; make appointment within 24 hours

Sign/Symptom	Observations	Associated Signs	Possible Condition	Action to Take
Gradual vision loss	Reluctant to go out at night. Bumps into walls/objects.	None	Cataracts (see Glossary). Retinal degeneration. Corneal degeneration. Corneal pigmentation.	See veterinarian
Sudden vision loss	Reluctant to move. Bumps into walls/objects.	None	Retinal degeneration. Retinal detachment. Intraocular hemorrhage. Acute glaucoma. Trauma.	See veterinarian
Red beanlike mass appears in corner of eye near nose	Usually young dog. Cockers and beagles more susceptible.	None	Cherry eye (swelling of gland of third eyelid—see p. 7)	See veterinarian. Medication rarely works. Surgery is usually recommended.
Brown streaks on fur below eyes (common in small poodles)	Chronically wet fur; eye overflows	None	Tear ducts abnormally formed or plugged	No treatment for mild cases. If problem is severe, ophthalmologist may be able to repair or relocate tear ducts.

Nuclear (Lenticular) Sclerosis

Almost all older dogs develop a bilateral cloudiness of the lenses of their eyes. An owner will first notice a gray or blue haze in certain lights, which may increase slightly as the dog ages. This is often confused with cataracts by owners, but a veterinary assessment will usually confirm that it is nuclear, or lenticular, sclerosis and is part of the normal aging process. As a dog ages, her lenses become cloudy and more dense. This condition does not significantly impair a dog's vision.

Call veterinarian; make appointment immediately

 Life-threatening condition; go *immediately* to veterinarian or emergency clinic

E
Y
E

D
I
S
O
R
D
E
R
S

External Genitalia (and Abnormal Discharges)

It is a good idea for an owner to examine a dog's external genital anatomy in order to know what it normally looks like. In a female, the only normal vulvar discharge is that associated with heat. The penis of a male dog is not usually visible. What is seen is a fur-covered sheath of skin that covers the penis. The penis itself may come out of the sheath when a dog is sexually excited or aroused.

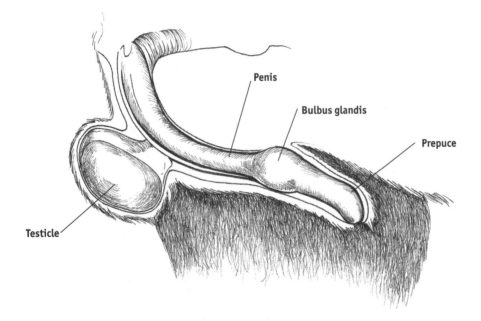

Side view of a dog's penis. Note that the penis is entirely enclosed by a sheath of skin unless the dog is sexually aroused.

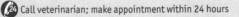

Home care; first aid   Call veterinarian   Call veterinarian; make appointment within 24 hours

Sign/Symptom	Observations	Associated Signs	Possible Condition	Action to Take
Swollen vulva	Dog attractive to male dogs	Mammary glands may be swollen. Pink or bloody vaginal discharge.	Heat period	✚ Do not allow access to male dogs for at least three weeks Consider spaying after heat period (see pp. 19–20)
Swollen vulva	May be depressed	Fever. Increased thirst and urination. Possible abdominal distension.	Nondraining pyometra (see p. 51)	(24) See veterinarian for X rays, blood work, surgery
Smelly mucoid or bloody vaginal discharge	Was recently in heat	Swollen vulva. Increased thirst and urination.	Draining pyometra (see p. 51; see also Box, below)	See veterinarian for X rays, blood work, surgery
Clear mucoid vaginal discharge	Young dog	None	Juvenile vaginal discharge	None needed. Will resolve in time, especially if spayed.

Pyometra *

A pyometra is a uterine infection, which is a very common condition in old, unspayed female dogs. It is one of the many reasons why female dogs should be spayed when young. In a closed pyometra, the pus builds up and the uterus distends like a sausage. In a draining pyometra, pus discharges from the vulva. There are medical approaches to the treatment of pyometra, but they are complex, expensive, and, generally, temporary. Surgical removal of the uterus is the correct approach in most cases. Pyometra is a serious medical problem that can be fatal if not treated appropriately.

*See also p. 51

 Call veterinarian; make appointment immediately   Life-threatening condition; go *immediately* to veterinarian or emergency clinic

Sign/Symptom	Observations	Associated Signs	Possible Condition	Action to Take
Yellow discharge from penis	Small amount of thick discharge may be left where dog was sleeping	None	Balanoposthitis—an infection of the sheath. Most unneutered male dogs have at least a bit of penile discharge.	➕ Usually none. If severe, see a veterinarian.
One testicle irregular or enlarged	Usually none	Possibly increased nipple size. Possibly attractive to male dogs. Other testicle may be atrophied (smaller).	Testicular tumor	🐾²⁴ See veterinarian for consultation, tests, possible castration
Swollen, painful testicle	Dog is reluctant to move, depressed	Possible fever	Infected testicle. Torsed (twisted within the scrotum) testicle.	🐾 See veterinarian for antibiotics or surgery
Penis is continually exposed	Penis may be red, swollen	Dog may lick at area	Paraphinosis (penis stuck out of sheath). Spinal problem.	🐾 See veterinarian if persistent

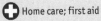 ➕ Home care; first aid   🐾 Call veterinarian   🐾²⁴ Call veterinarian; make appointment within 24 hours

Gagging

Gagging implies a throat problem and should not be confused with coughing, which comes from lower down in the airways. When the throat is inflamed for any reason, a gag reflex ensues. Dogs often gag up mucus and swallow it. Other times, small amounts of mucus, or white foam, is spit out. If the foam is bloody, there is usually an infection, foreign object, or bleeding mass in the throat.

Sign/Symptom	Observations	Associated Signs	Possible Condition	Action to Take
Acute gagging	Coughs before or after, may bring up small amounts of mucoid white foam	None. May also sneeze.	"Kennel cough" (see pp. 59–60). Pharyngitis/tonsillitis.	See veterinarian for cough suppressants, other medication
Acute gagging	Vomits. Regurgitates food or saliva.	Salivates excessively.	Plant ingestion (see Appendix A, pp. 157–58). Chemical ingestion (see Appendix A). Esophagitis. Foreign body in the esophagus.	Withhold food and water Go to the emergency clinic for treatment
Chronic gagging	Cough precedes gagging. May also have noisy breathing.	Becomes worse with excitement or in warm weather	Collapsing trachea. Laryngeal paralysis.	See veterinarian for X rays
Episodic gagging	Snorts/gasps	Clear nasal discharge	Reverse sneeze (see Box, p. 139). Post-nasal drip. Allergies.	See veterinarian for evaluation
Progressive, chronic gagging	Possible swollen neck	Difficulty swallowing. Weight loss.	Thyroid cancer. Tonsillar cancer. Swollen lymph nodes. Abscess. Foreign object in back of throat.	Go to emergency clinic for examination, X rays, biopsy

 Call veterinarian; make appointment immediately

 Life-threatening condition; go *immediately* to veterinarian or emergency clinic

Sign/Symptom	Observations	Associated Signs	Possible Condition	Action to Take
Acute or chronic gagging	Painful neck or throat	Possible fever. Gags up white or bloody mucus.	Abscess. Possible foreign body, such as a needle, in throat.	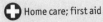 See veterinarian for examination, possible X rays

 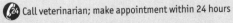

Incoordination

Dogs that are incoordinated will wobble when walking, and their legs may cross over each other. Sometimes they will also drag their feet. This usually occurs in all four legs but it may be confined to the rear legs. Incoordinated dogs do not improve with exercise, as opposed to arthritic dogs, which often become less stiff after moving around.

Sign/Symptom	Observations	Associated Signs	Possible Condition	Action to Take
Rear legs incoordinated	Slowly progressive	May have back pain	Spinal cord tumor. Degenerative spinal cord disease (especially in German shepherds). Spinal disc disease. Instability of cervical vertebrae (especially in Dobermans and Great Danes).	Consult veterinarian for X rays and treatment
Rear legs incoordinated	Rapid onset	May have back pain	Acute spinal disc disease. Spinal cord trauma.	Go to emergency clinic for X rays
All four legs incoordinated	Slowly progressive	May have neck pain	Cervical spinal cord disc, instability, or tumor	See veterinarian for X rays
All four legs incoordinated	Progressive	May have personality changes, seizures, fever	Brain tumor. Inflammatory brain disease (encephalitis) (see Glossary).	Go to emergency clinic immediately

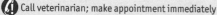 Call veterinarian; make appointment immediately

 Life-threatening condition; go *immediately* to veterinarian or emergency clinic

Sign/Symptom	Observations	Associated Signs	Possible Condition	Action to Take
All four legs incoordinated	Rapid onset	Vomiting and/or diarrhea. Depression. Possible seizures.	Poisoning (see pp. 47–48; 55; Appendix A, pp. 157–58). Head trauma. Rarely, vascular insult to brain.	✚ If poisoned, try to determine what was ingested—this is invaluable information ⚠ Go to emergency clinic, or call ASPCA National Animal Poison Control Center, 800-548-2423
Incoordination	Doesn't want to move. Falls to one side.	Head tilt; eyeballs twitch; vomiting; anorexia	Inner/middle ear disease or infection. Idiopathic canine vestibular syndrome. Brain tumor.	✚ May give veterinarian-approved medication for nausea. Protect dog from falling downstairs. ☎ Consult veterinarian for examination, possible X rays

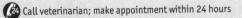

✚ Home care; first aid   ☎ Call veterinarian   🕑 Call veterinarian; make appointment within 24 hours

L

Lameness

Lameness is a condition that can have many causes. It can arise due to a simple twisted joint, similar to a sprained ankle in humans, or it may have a deeper underlying cause. It can also stem from a sore paw, irritated by snow-removal chemicals, a foreign object stuck between the toes, or a laceration of a footpad.

A dog is lame if she changes her gait to shift weight and make it less painful to use her leg. First, determine which leg she is favoring. If she holds it up, it is obvious, but if not, try to determine which leg she puts the least weight on when standing. Watch her walk. When a front leg is lame, a dog will often "head bob"—that is, her head will go up when weight is placed on the leg that is hurting.

If it can be determined which leg is bothering the dog, the leg should be examined thoroughly. (If the dog is aggressive and/or in a great deal of pain, be careful not to be bitten—it may be best to leave the examination to a veterinarian.) Starting at the foot, squeeze each toe separately and then the entire foot. Work up the leg, squeezing gently. It may be possible to locate the area of pain, but this is often not successful, however, and X rays may be required to make a definite diagnosis.

Lameness is rarely an emergency, unless it is accompanied by extreme pain or an obvious fracture. Sprains and strains usually get better given time and patience.

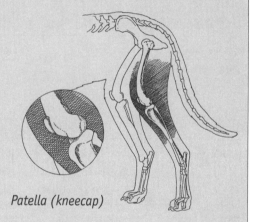

Patella (kneecap)

Sign/Symptom	Observations	Associated Signs	Possible Condition	Action to Take
All four legs painful	Does not want to walk	Possible fever. Possible swollen joints.	Polyarthropathy; (see Glossary). Lyme disease (see p. 62); arthritis; myositis (inflamed muscles). Young large-breed dogs, hypertrophic osteodystrophy (HOD) (see Glossary).	See veterinarian for tests

 Call veterinarian; make appointment immediately

Life-threatening condition; go *immediately* to veterinarian or emergency clinic

Sign/Symptom	Observations	Associated Signs	Possible Condition	Action to Take
Lame in one front leg	Progressive or sudden	Neck pain. May hold one leg up.	Cervical lesion, caused by a disc, tumor, or trauma	See veterinarian for X rays, medication
Lame on any one leg	Progressive. Large-breed dog, middle age or older.	Leg swelling	Bone tumor	See veterinarian for X rays
Lame on foreleg	Episodic or progressive. Young, large-breed dog.	None	Developmental bone or cartilage defect (i.e., OCD—osteochondritis dissecans; elbow dysplasia; ununited coronoid process; etc.)	See veterinarian for examination and X rays
Sudden-onset lameness in one leg	May lick foot	None	Toe problem: fractured/dislocated toe; cut toe; torn/broken nail	First aid if cut See veterinarian for X ray, or to remove broken nail
Painful hips	Somewhat chronic. Large-breed dog. Slow getting up.	None	Hip dysplasia	See veterinarian for medication and/or X rays
Stiff rear legs, improves with exercise	Progressive. Older dog. Has trouble going up stairs.	None	Arthritis in any or all joints	See veterinarian for medication and/or X rays
Episodic lameness in one rear leg	Small-breed dog. Will go from normal to holding leg up, back to normal. Lameness will get better if leg is pulled straight down.	None	Luxating patella (kneecap)	See veterinarian. Some small dogs become acclimated to the patella moving in and out of place and need no treatment. Some require surgery.

Home care; first aid   Call veterinarian   Call veterinarian; make appointment within 24 hours

Sign/Symptom	Observations	Associated Signs	Possible Condition	Action to Take
One rear leg acutely lame	May have cried once, then held leg up	None	Ruptured cranial cruciate ligament in the knee (cruciate ligaments keep knees stable)	See veterinarian for X rays, possible surgery
Lame on one or both rear legs	Reluctant to move	Painful back	Lumbar disc disease; tumor; trauma	See veterinarian for X rays and/or medication
Lame on one rear leg	Progressive. Young, small-breed dog.	None	Aseptic necrosis of femoral head (degeneration of ball part of femur, or thigh bone, also called Legg-Calvé-Perthes disease)	See veterinarian for X rays and surgery
Lame on any one leg or lameness that shifts from one leg to another	Young, large-breed, growing dog	Possible fever, lethargy	Panosteitis	See veterinarian for X rays

Toenails

Abnormal toenails may cause lameness under certain circumstances. If a nail is cracked or partially broken off, there is pain and lameness. Dogs may have nails that grow in circles and become ingrown, causing pain. There are also bacterial, fungal, and immune-mediated diseases that affect nails, causing pain.

Care of a dog's nails should, to a great extent, be determined by the individual dog. Dogs that are shown must have their nails clipped very short. Dogs whose nails tend to become ingrown or break easily should have nails trimmed regularly. Owners often complain that their dog scratches people, and attempt to alleviate this by cutting the dog's nails very short. It is better to train the dog not to jump up on people. Many dogs do not need regular nail trims. Their nails become worn down by exercise. If a dog has dew claws, they need to be watched carefully because they are higher on the leg and are not worn down. Dew claws can grow into the foot, break, or become caught in blankets or rugs.

 Call veterinarian; make appointment immediately

 Life-threatening condition; go *immediately* to veterinarian or emergency clinic

Mammary Gland Abnormalities

Dogs have ten mammary glands, five on each side. Each has a corresponding nipple that is fairly small in males and in females that are not nursing. In both sexes, the nipples are sometimes confused with small skin masses by owners. Female mammary glands are barely visible until after the first heat period. The size varies with individuals and hormonal changes after the first heat. As we mentioned in Chapter 2 (see "Spaying and Neutering," pages 19–20), females spayed before their first heat period have virtually no chance of developing breast cancer. There is a significant reduction in risk if spaying occurs between the first and second heat periods. Any female dog that has gone through heat periods should be regularly examined for breast masses.

Sign/Symptom	Observations	Associated Signs	Possible Condition	Action to Take
Breast tissue enlarging fairly rapidly	Just completed heat cycle	None	Normal development	None
Breast tissue enlarged	Intact female. Was in heat approximately two months previously.	Abdomen enlarged (see also Abdominal Distension). *Milk in mammary glands.* Increased appetite.	Pregnancy	🐾 See veterinarian for diagnosis
Breast tissue enlarged	Was in heat about two months ago. Was not bred.	Milk in mammary glands without abdominal enlargement	False pregnancy	None. Normally resolves itself. 🐾 If severe personality changes occur, may need to spay or take medication
One or more mammary glands enlarged, hot, and painful	Usually nursing bitch. Milk from that gland abnormal color.	Fever. Lethargy.	Mastitis (bacterial infection of mammary gland)	🐾 See veterinarian for antibiotics and treatment

➕ Home care; first aid   🐾 Call veterinarian   🐾24 Call veterinarian; make appointment within 24 hours

Sign/Symptom	Observations	Associated Signs	Possible Condition	Action to Take
Multiple small masses in breast tissue	May have recently gone through heat period	None	Multiple cysts (could be tumors)	See veterinarian for opinion, possible biopsy, possible surgery
Small or large growing masses in breast tissue	Has had previous heat periods	None	Breast tumors	See veterinarian for biopsy/surgical removal. Possible spay.
Male dog, enlarged nipples	Dog attractive to other males	Possible change in size or feel of testicles (see also External Genitalia)	Sertoli cell tumor (estrogen-secreting tumor) of testicle	See veterinarian for castration

M
A
M
M
A
R
Y

G
L
A
N
D

A
B
N
O
R
M
A
L
I
T
I
E
S

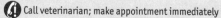 Call veterinarian; make appointment immediately   Life-threatening condition; go *immediately* to veterinarian or emergency clinic

Mouth Disorders

An owner who brushes her dog's teeth on a regular basis (see pages 26–27) will probably detect mouth problems before they become too serious. An owner who does not routinely perform tooth brushing should examine her dog's mouth from time to time, looking at the teeth, along the gum lines, and underneath the tongue for any redness, swelling, or other abnormalities. The most common external signs associated with oral lesions are foul odor and drooling. However, bad breath is not always associated with a mouth problem, but may be one sign of an underlying systemic disease. For example, the odor of waste products on a dog's breath may be a sign of kidney disease or sweet, fruity breath may indicate diabetes mellitus.

Sign/Symptom	Observations	Associated Signs	Possible Condition	Action to Take
Drooling, bad breath	May spit out food	Possible bloody saliva	Bad teeth: abscessed tooth; severe dental disease with loose, painful teeth	🕐24 See veterinarian for dentistry
Bad breath	Older dog. Slowly becoming worse.	Drooling. Possible swelling of jaw or face.	Oral tumor	🕐 See veterinarian for tests, biopsy, possible surgery
Pawing at mouth	Rapid onset. May not eat. Uncomfortable.	Possible drooling	Foreign body caught across roof of mouth or on tooth. Loose tooth that has shifted in mouth.	➕ Look at roof of mouth and remove object 🕐 If loose tooth, see veterinarian for removal. See also Appetite, Abnormal, pp. 95–97.

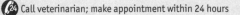

➕ Home care; first aid   🕐 Call veterinarian   🕐24 Call veterinarian; make appointment within 24 hours

Dental Disease

The most common oral problems in dogs are related to tartar formation and subsequent gum recession. All dogs develop a certain amount of tartar. How fast it develops is a function of several things. Veterinarians will agree that genetic predisposition is probably the most important factor. Small-breed dogs are overrepresented in the "bad teeth" category. Diet can also play a role—the harder and more abrasive the food in the diet, the more slowly tartar will form. Special abrasive diets have been developed to slow down tartar formation. In addition, there are many types of artificial bones and chew toys that can help reduce tartar formation (giving real bones can be potentially dangerous and is not recommended). The single most important thing an owner can do to help promote healthy teeth and gums and slow down tartar development is to brush a dog's teeth—see pages 26–27—or have the teeth professionally cleaned on a regular basis.

When tartar builds up and causes gum disease, it is more than just aesthetically unpleasant. There is evidence that gum disease may lead to problems in a dog's kidneys or heart.

Periodically, the veterinarian may suggest that a dog needs a dental cleaning and polishing under anesthetic. Loose teeth may also need to be extracted. There are veterinarians who are board certified in dentistry. They can perform more difficult dentistry, such as root canals, periodontal work, tooth restoration, and orthodontia.

 Call veterinarian; make appointment immediately   ⊞ Life-threatening condition; go *immediately* to veterinarian or emergency clinic

Sign/Symptom	Observations	Associated Signs	Possible Condition	Action to Take
Bad breath	Slowly progressive. Dog may be losing weight.	Depressed appetite. Nausea. Vomiting. Increased thirst.	Kidney dysfunction	🕓 See veterinarian for tests. Bring urine sample.
Baby teeth do not fall out	Usually canine teeth of small dogs not out by six months of age	None	Retained deciduous (baby) teeth	📞 See veterinarian for removal. Retained teeth trap food, causing tartar and shifting of adult canines.
Dog cannot close lower jaw	Has difficulty eating and drinking	Drools	Nerve dysfunction affecting the trigeminal nerve— usually idiopathic (of no known cause)	➕ If rabies possible, go to emergency clinic 📞 If idiopathic, eventually resolves with supportive food and fluids
Flat black areas apparent on gums or tongue	None	None	Normal pigment change	None
Dog cannot open mouth	Usually progressive, rapid onset	Cannot eat or drink	Myositis of chewing muscles	🕓 See veterinarian for treatment, possible surgery
Severe jaw pain in young terrier dog	Progressive	May have difficulty eating; cries when touched	Craniomandibular osteopathy	📞 See veterinarian for X rays, treatment

➕ Home care; first aid   📞 Call veterinarian   🕓 Call veterinarian; make appointment within 24 hours

Mucous Membrane Color

One of the best ways to ascertain the condition of a dog is to examine his mucous membranes. The easiest and quickest way to do this is to lift the dog's upper lip to see the gums and cheeks. Normally, a dog's interior mouth tissues are a bright pink. Changes in color to bright red, pale pink, white, yellow, orange, blue, or purple usually indicate serious medical problems. In some breeds, however, gums and other interior mouth tissues are normally black or dark purple. In these cases the inside of the vagina or penile sheath or the interior eyelids are the only places to see normal mucous membrane pigmentation. It is a good idea to examine a dog's mucous membranes when he is well in order to assess an abnormal condition if necessary.

Sign/Symptom	Observations	Associated Signs	Possible Condition	Action to Take
Bright-red membranes	Could act normal. Depression/lethargy.	Convulsions. Increased thirst, urination (polydipsia; polyuria)	Polycythemia (see Glossary)	Call the veterinarian for fluids, tests. If convulsions, go immediately to emergency clinic
Brick-red membranes	Seriously depressed. Weak. Lethargic.	Fever	Severe bacterial infection	Go to emergency clinic for fluids, tests, medication
Blue/purple membranes	Difficult/labored breathing	Collapse. Weakness.	Heart failure (see "Cardiovascular Emergencies," pp. 49–50). Serious respiratory disease (see "Breathing Problems," p. 49). Respiratory obstruction.	Go to emergency clinic for X rays, medication

 Call veterinarian; make appointment immediately   Life-threatening condition; go *immediately* to veterinarian or emergency clinic

Sign/Symptom	Observations	Associated Signs	Possible Condition	Action to Take
Yellow/orange membranes	Whites of eyes, skin, appear yellow	Vomiting. Diarrhea. Appetite loss. Abdominal pain.	Liver disease. Pancreatitis. Jaundice (see Glossary). Hemolytic anemia (see "anemia," Glossary). Gall bladder disease.	🕿 Call the veterinarian for tests, medication
Pale pink/white membranes	Weak. Unable to rise. Seriously depressed. Unresponsive.	Possible black stools. Possible external hemorrhage.	Shock (see Box, p. 53). Addison's disease (see Glossary). Anemia. Internal hemorrhage. Heart failure (see "Cardiovascular Emergencies," pp. 49–50). Rat poison ingestion (see "Poisoning," pp. 47–48; see also Appendix A, pp. 157–58). Bleeding disorder (see pp. 48–49). Severe dehydration (see Box, p. 152).	❗ Go to emergency clinic for tests, possible transfusion, medication
Pale pink/white mucous membranes	Tires easily. Lethargic.	Possible black stools. Pica (see Glossary).	Anemia. Fleas. Worms. Zinc toxicity (ingestion of pennies). Rat poison (see "Poisoning," pp. 47–48; see also Appendix A, pp. 157–58).	🕿24 to ❗ See veterinarian for X rays, tests, medication, possible transfusion. The more lethargic, the more serious.

➕ Home care; first aid   🕿 Call veterinarian   🕿24 Call veterinarian; make appointment within 24 hours

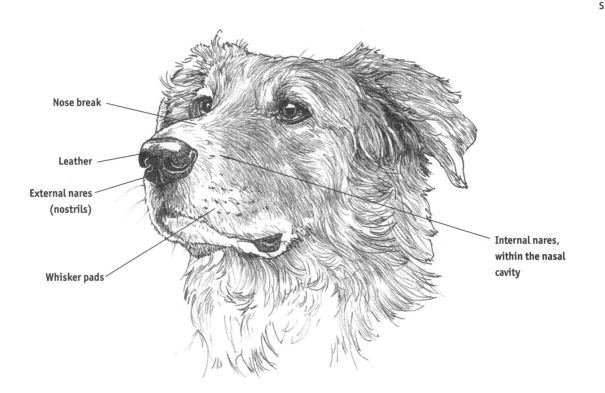

Nasal Disorders,
Including Changes in the Nares

There are a number of nasal disorders that are characterized by a discharge, either bloody, mucoid, or purulent. Sometimes a diagnosis can be made by flushing fluid into the dog's nose and examining the fluid retrieved. Often it is necessary for a dog to be anesthetized so the veterinarian can use a nasoscope to evaluate the upper nasal area for a diagnosis. A CT (CAT) scan (see Glossary) or MRI (see Glossary), if available, is extremely useful in both diagnosis and prognosis.

Nose break

Leather

External nares
(nostrils)

Whisker pads

Internal nares,
within the nasal
cavity

A Dog's Nose

 Call veterinarian; make appointment immediately

Life-threatening condition; go *immediately* to veterinarian
or emergency clinic

Sign/Symptom	Observations	Associated Signs	Possible Condition	Action to Take
Bilateral or unilateral bloody, purulent (pussy), or mucoid nasal discharge	Chronic, usually progressive	Sneezing	Nasal tumor. Foreign body in nose. Nasal infection, bacterial or fungal. Sinusitis.	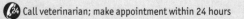 See veterinarian for tests, X rays
Bloody discharge, both sides	May have tiny skin or gum hemorrhages	May be bleeding elsewhere	Clotting problem due to: drugs (see "Drug Poisoning/ Intoxication," p. 55); rat poison ingestion (see "Poisoning," pp. 47–48; Appendix A, pp. 157–58); ehrlichiosis (see "Canine Ehrlichiosis," p. 61); immune-mediated problem	Go to emergency clinic for laboratory tests
Bloody nose	Sneezing a lot	Usually none	Broken blood vessel secondary to sneezing, trauma, or foreign object	See veterinarian. Sedation may help. Try to stop sneezing with veterinarian-recommended antihistamine or cortisone
Black nares become pink	Occurred slowly	None	Very common, especially in light-coated dogs. Unlikely a medical cause. May be genetic.	None

Home care; first aid　　　Call veterinarian　　　Call veterinarian; make appointment within 24 hours

Sign/Symptom	Observations	Associated Signs	Possible Condition	Action to Take
Nose becomes scabby and ulcerated	Older, possibly light-colored dog. Slowly progressive.	None	Tumor, usually squamous cell carcinoma (see Glossary)	See veterinarian for biopsy and possible surgery, radiation
Nares become scabby and ulcerated	Often collies and collie-mix dogs; also Shetland sheepdogs, others. Some spotty loss of pigment. Might be worse after sun exposure.	Usually none	"Collie nose." Discoid lupus (form of autoimmune disease).	See veterinarian for steroids, sunscreen, possible vitamin E
Nasal openings very small	Usually brachycephalic breeds (see Glossary). May tire with exercise. Poor heat tolerance.	Snorting	Congenital problem	See veterinarian for minor surgery, which may help prevent future problems
Snoring	Usually slowly progressive	Common in brachycephalic breeds	Decrease in tone of throat tissue. Obstruction (tumor) in throat.	See veterinarian to eliminate possibility of mass in throat. Severe snoring may be helped with surgery.
Swelling of nose	Acute onset. May or may not be symmetrical.	Rubs at face	Allergic reaction to insect bite or food	✚ Veterinary-recommended antihistamine or cortisone See veterinarian if very uncomfortable or does not resolve

N
A
S
A
L

D
I
S
O
R
D
E
R
S

 Call veterinarian; make appointment immediately ✚ Life-threatening condition; go *immediately* to veterinarian or emergency clinic

Sign/Symptom	Observations	Associated Signs	Possible Condition	Action to Take
Swelling on top of or along bridge of nose	Usually older dog. Growing slowly.	Sneezing. Nasal discharge.	Tumor	See veterinarian for X rays, other tests. Surgery may be recommended but is often not curative, even when combined with chemotherapy or radiation.
Swelling below eye	May be draining blood or pus	Possible fever	Abscessed fourth premolar tooth	See veterinarian for antibiotics and tooth extraction

Rectal Problems

There may be signs such as swelling or redness when a dog has a problem with his rectum. Often, however, there is no external evidence of a problem, except that the dog's rectum seems to be itching. This is usually indicated by excessive licking, or by "scooting"—that is, sliding or dragging the rear end on the floor.

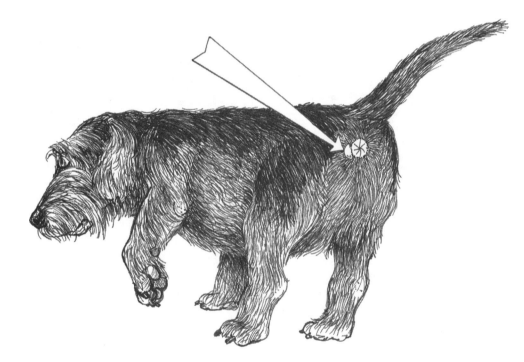

Impacted anal sac

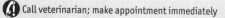 Call veterinarian; make appointment immediately

 Life-threatening condition; go *immediately* to veterinarian or emergency clinic

Sign/Symptom	Observations	Associated Signs	Possible Condition	Action to Take
One or more masses around the rectum	Unaltered male dog. Masses grow slowly, may bleed.	Licking to clean blood	Perianal (see Glossary) adenoma (usually a benign tumor)	See veterinarian for removal, possible hormonal therapy, possible castration
Firm swelling around rectum, progressive	May have difficulty moving bowels	None	Tumor, either rectal or internal	See veterinarian for examination, tests, biopsy, possible surgery
Soft swelling to side of rectum	Unaltered male. Difficulty moving bowels.	None	Perineal (see Glossary) hernia	See veterinarian for examination, hernia repair, castration
Scooting on rectum	Small (half-inch) off-white worm segments on stool	None	Tapeworms	See veterinarian for medication, flea control. (Note: This is a rare reason for scooting. Tapeworms are the only worms that cause rectal itch in dogs. Dogs do not get pinworms.)

Home care; first aid Call veterinarian Call veterinarian; make appointment within 24 hours

Sign/Symptom	Observations	Associated Signs	Possible Condition	Action to Take
Scooting on rectum	May be sporadic or progressive	Licking at rectum. May notice foul odor.	Anal sac infection/impaction	See veterinarian to express or infuse sacs ✚ In case of impacted sacs, owners may learn to express sacs. High-fiber diet may help keep sacs empty. (Note: If chronic, anal sacs may be removed.)
Red, purple swelling to side of rectum	May be lethargic. May strain to move bowels.	Fever. Bloody discharge from area if ruptured.	Anal sac abscess	See veterinarian for antibiotics and possible drainage
Excessive tail chasing	None	None	Behavioral. May be compulsive behavior.	See veterinarian to discuss medical options

R

E
C
T
A
L

P
R
O
B
L
E
M
S

Respiratory Difficulties

Respiratory difficulties include both problems that cause labored or difficult breathing (dyspnea), and those that cause coughing. (See boxes for panting and reverse sneezing, opposite and p.139). Labored breathing need not be rapid, but it is abnormal in that a dog requires more effort than usual to inhale or exhale. A dog whose breathing is labored will use his stomach muscles to help him get enough air.

Coughing is a very common nonspecific sign, and should not be confused with *gagging* or *reverse sneezing*. The type of cough, severity, and other associated signs indicate the significance of a cough.

A dog with severe respiratory difficulties should not be exercised or subjected to a hot environment. A blue or purplish color to mucous membranes indicates a severe, life-threatening emergency.

Sign/Symptom	Observations	Associated Signs	Possible Condition	Action to Take
Labored breathing	Dog is not moving much; does not want to lie down	Cough. Tongue may appear purple. Nasal discharge.	If nasal discharge is mucoid—pneumonia. If nasal discharge is foamy white—cardiac failure (see "Cardiovascular Emergencies," pp. 49–50), or electrocution (see p. 55).	Go to emergency clinic immediately
Labored breathing	Dog lethargic. May not want to lie down.	Cough. Bluish (cyanotic) tongue.	Cardiac failure (see "Cardiovascular Emergencies," pp. 49–50). Lung tumor. Obstruction of trachea. Pneumonia. Trauma to lungs accompanied by bleeding or swelling.	Go to emergency clinic immediately

Home care; first aid   Call veterinarian   Call veterinarian; make appointment within 24 hours

Sign/Symptom	Observations	Associated Signs	Possible Condition	Action to Take
Labored breathing	Dog weak	Pale mucous membranes	Anemia. Shock (see Box, p. 53).	⊕ Go to emergency clinic immediately
Labored breathing	History of trauma to chest (e.g., hit by car)	May be in pain or have cuts/scratches indicating some type of trauma	Fluid or blood in lungs. Collapsed lung. Air in chest cavity (pneumothorax). Diaphragmatic hernia (abdominal organs move through ruptured diaphragm into chest cavity).	⊕ Go to emergency clinic immediately
Labored breathing	Dog lethargic. May not want to lie down.	None. No cough.	Pleural effusion (fluid in chest around the lungs). Chest tumor.	⊕ Go to emergency clinic immediately
Cough	Poor exercise tolerance. Cough becoming progressively worse.	May cough up mucus, or yellow or green pus. May also have labored breathing and mucoid nasal discharge.	Pneumonia.	Take temperature (see pp. 70–71) ⓘ If temperature is normal and dog stable, see the veterinarian ⊕ If temperature is over 103, go to emergency clinic immediately

Panting

Panting is shallow, rapid, open-mouth breathing usually not associated with true medical problems. Dogs normally pant when they are hot, nervous, or excited. However, dogs taking cortisone may pant, and dogs often pant when they are in pain. If a dog exhibits constant, unexplained panting, a veterinary opinion should be sought.

ⓘ Call veterinarian; make appointment immediately

⊕ Life-threatening condition; go *immediately* to veterinarian or emergency clinic

Sign/Symptom	Observations	Associated Signs	Possible Condition	Action to Take
Cough	Lethargic. Cough mostly nocturnal, progressively worsening.	May have labored breathing. May have bluish mucous membranes (cyanosis). May have frothy nasal discharge. May faint.	Cardiac failure (see "Cardiovascular Emergencies," pp. 49–50)	(24) If no associated symptoms are present, see the veterinarian (!) If any associated symptoms are present, go to emergency clinic immediately
Cough	Fairly rapid onset. Harsh, honking cough, especially when pulling on leash.	May also gag up white foam	Kennel cough (see pp. 59–60). Tracheal disease. Tracheal collapse, especially adult toy dogs.	(+) If kennel cough suspected, may use veterinarian-recommended over-the-counter pediatric cough syrups (24) If not responsive to cough syrups, see the veterinarian
Chronic cough	Sometimes coughs up mucus	None	Chronic bronchitis, allergic bronchitis. Bronchitis in dogs is often related to tracheal collapse. Secondary to irritant.	(call) See veterinarian for X rays, medication, possible tests
Difficulty inhaling	Often brachycephalic breeds. Noise comes from nose and throat. Tires with exercise. Poor heat tolerance.	Possibly cyanotic (see Glossary)	Elongated soft palate. Obstruction of larynx (tumor, foreign body).	(call) If chronic, see veterinarian for diagnosis and possible surgery (!) If onset is acute and foreign body suspected, go to emergency clinic immediately

(+) Home care; first aid   (call) Call veterinarian   (24) Call veterinarian; make appointment within 24 hours

Reverse Sneezing

Because this is not a human action, owners have difficulty describing what happens. It seems to be an asthmatic attack, or the inability of a dog to catch his breath. It sounds as if the dog is repeatedly snorting. In reality, it is a series of spasmodic, rapid inhalations through the nose. Dogs usually go from acting perfectly normal to having an episode of reverse sneezing that lasts for about thirty seconds. The dog then returns to acting normal.

Reverse sneezing is caused by an irritation in the pharynx. Anything that causes irritation in the pharynx will trigger an attack. Normally, it is associated with allergies or sore throats and is more common in brachycephalic breeds. Often, feeding a dog soft foods will alleviate the problem. If it becomes severe, the veterinarian may prescribe anti-inflammatory drugs and antibiotics.

 Call veterinarian; make appointment immediately   Life-threatening condition; go *immediately* to veterinarian or emergency clinic

Skin Disorders

This is an extremely broad category. The areas covered include: changes in haircoat; bumps, lumps, and swelling; infections; parasitic diseases; rashes, color changes, and causes of itching (pruritis).

The underlying causes of skin problems can be very difficult to diagnose. There are veterinarians who specialize in dermatology who may be consulted in very difficult or persistent cases.

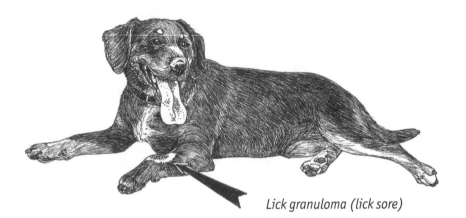

Lick granuloma (lick sore)

Ticks

(See also "Fleas and Ticks," page 26)

Owners sometimes confuse an engorged female tick with a skin tumor. Male brown dog ticks and nonengorged females are small, brown, and flat (about an eighth of an inch in diameter). Females fill up with blood as they feed and look like green-gray beans about a quarter to a half inch long. There are four small legs on each side, near the mouth parts. Ticks may be removed from a dog with tweezers. It is not usually a problem if a small portion of the mouth parts remains in the skin; it will come out on its own. Ticks do not burrow beneath the skin. The deer tick responsible for Lyme disease transmission is much smaller than the common brown dog tick. Even engorged, they may be difficult to find.

Home care; first aid   Call veterinarian   Call veterinarian; make appointment within 24 hours

Sign/Symptom	Observations	Associated Signs	Possible Condition	Action to Take
Hair coming out in clumps	Double-coated dog. Normal coat underneath lost hair.	None	Shedding undercoat	✚ Groom frequently (see "Grooming and Bathing," pp. 24–27)
Symmetrical hair loss, mostly on the trunk of the body	Hair brittle/dull. Possibly lethargic. Possibly averse to cold.	Skin may become darker	Hypothyroidism	🐾 See veterinarian for endocrine tests and medication
Hair thinning on sides/abdomen	Increased appetite, thirst, and urination	Pot belly	Cushing's syndrome (see Glossary)	🐾 See veterinarian for blood tests
Areas of hair loss, usually around eyes and face	Young dog	None	Localized demodectic mange (caused by the Demodex canis mite)	🐾 See veterinarian for skin scraping and treatment
Facial swelling	May rub or paw at face	None	Allergic reaction, usually to food or an insect bite	✚ Give veterinarian-approved antihistamines or cortisone 🐾 See veterinarian if not resolved
Multiple raised areas on skin. Acute onset.	Usually on head. May be itchy.	None	Hives due to an acute allergy	✚ Give veterinarian-approved antihistamines or cortisone 🐾 See veterinarian if not resolved
Growing lumps	Usually slow-growing. May be soft, firm, or irregular.	None	Cysts or tumors	🐾 See veterinarian for examination, possible biopsy, possible removal
Multiple masses on skin	Skin may be scabby or greasy. Irregular surface. Dog middle-aged or older. Common in poodles.	Possibly itchy	Sebaceous gland adenomas (normally benign skin tumors)	🐾 Discuss treatment with veterinarian

🐾 Call veterinarian; make appointment immediately   ❗ Life-threatening condition; go *immediately* to veterinarian or emergency clinic

S

K
I
N

D
I
S
O
R
D
E
R
S

Sign/Symptom	Observations	Associated Signs	Possible Condition	Action to Take
Lumps, usually on neck	Lumps may also be felt in groin, behind knees, in front of shoulder. Dog may be depressed.	Usually none, initially	Swollen lymph nodes. Lymphoma (cancer of the lymph nodes). Inflammation of the lymph nodes. Systemic disease.	🐾24 See veterinarian for biopsy or tests
Swelling below eye— see Nasal Disorders				
Swelling to side of rectum—see Rectal Problems				
Swelling of mammary glands—see Mammary Gland Abnormalities				
Patchy hair loss	May be itchy	Possibly scabs, crusts, small abscesses, or pus	Bacterial skin disease, or demodectic mange with secondary bacterial infection	🐾 See veterinarian for skin scraping, tests, medication
Patchy hair loss	Usually round in shape	Usually not itchy	Ringworm (a fungal infection)	🐾 See veterinarian for diagnosis, culture, and treatment. Ringworm may be contagious to humans and other pets.
Bloody discharge between some toes	Swollen, discolored tissue normally between several toes. May be on different feet. Often seen in German shepherds and spaniels.	None	Interdigital abscesses (bacterial disease with possible allergic component)	🐾 See veterinarian for antibiotics and possible drainage

✚ Home care; first aid   🐾 Call veterinarian   🐾24 Call veterinarian; make appointment within 24 hours

Sign/Symptom	Observations	Associated Signs	Possible Condition	Action to Take
Solitary area swollen, red, painful	May be draining pus	Possible fever	Abscess, or infected cyst or tumor	See veterinarian for diagnosis, antibiotics. May need drainage or surgical removal.
Acute appearance of weepy, painful area	May be large or small. Usually on rump or head. May be obviously infected and smelly.	If large, dog may be depressed	Hot spot; also called moist eczema, superficial dermatitis	See veterinarian to clip, give antibiotics, possibly steroids. May need to use an Elizabethan collar (see p. 70)
Dog chronically itchy	Scratches at body, rubs face, chews feet and legs	May produce scabs and secondary bacterial infections	Allergy (inhaled, food, contact; usually adult dogs). Sarcoptic mange (scabies; usually young dogs).	See veterinarian for tests or medication
Chronic licking of area on lower foreleg or back leg	Area becomes raised and ulcerated	None	Lick granuloma (Acral lick dermatitis) (see Glossary).	See veterinarian to discuss options, which include: medical treatment; behavioral assessment; possibly acupuncture

Call veterinarian; make appointment immediately   Life-threatening condition; go *immediately* to veterinarian or emergency clinic

Sign/Symptom	Observations	Associated Signs	Possible Condition	Action to Take
Hair loss and itching on the rump and back legs	Generally uncomfortable	None	Flea bite allergy	🕐24 See veterinarian for flea control (see "Fleas and Ticks," p. 26), cortisone, antihistamines, possible antibiotics

(Note: It only takes one flea bite every several days to perpetuate this condition. It does not necessarily indicate a severe infestation of fleas. Fleas may, in fact, be hard to find, but flea dirt is usually evident. All fleas on all pets, and in the environment, must be eradicated.)

Sign/Symptom	Observations	Associated Signs	Possible Condition	Action to Take
Scattered hemorrhages or bruises on skin	None	May bleed from anywhere (gums, nose, in urine or stool)	Clotting defect, caused by: rat poison; drugs (see Poisoning, pp. 47–48; see also Appendix A, pp. 157–58); DIC (see Glossary); immune-mediated thrombocytopenia, systemic lupus erythematosus (see Glossary); other.	⊕ Go to emergency clinic for tests
Skin becoming darker	Possibly lethargic	Possible hair loss	Hormonal imbalance (usually hypothyroid). May be genetic.	📞 See veterinarian for blood tests, possible biopsy
Solitary mass with hole in middle	None	None	Fly larva developing under skin, abscess	📞 See veterinarian for treatment

S

K
I
N

D
I
S
O
R
D
E
R
S

Dietary Influence on Coat

There are clearly nutritional elements for a proper coat. Although we may not know every one, or the nutritional requirements of an individual dog, high-quality commercial and "designer" foods are excellent for most dogs. Certain diets, or homemade diets, may be deficient in vitamins, minerals, or essential fats. Sometimes a dog has difficulty absorbing the proper nutritional elements from a complete diet. If a dog's coat is not good, and medical explanations have been reasonably eliminated, look at the dog's diet. A diet change to a higher quality, higher nutrient food may help.

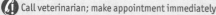
Call veterinarian; make appointment immediately   Life-threatening condition; go *immediately* to veterinarian or emergency clinic

Straining to Move Bowels

When a dog strains to move her bowels, it is usually associated with constipation by most owners. In fact, many dogs that have to strain to move their bowels have colitis (inflammation of the colon). When a dog is straining to move her bowels, the form of the stool determines if it is constipation (hard stools), or colitis (small amounts of mucoid stool, sometimes bloody). Dogs rarely have primary constipation. When they are chronically constipated, it is commonly due to a disease of the colon, anus, or perianal area.

Sign/Symptom	Observations	Associated Signs	Possible Condition	Action to Take
Straining to move bowels	Frequently stops, squats, strains. Acute or chronic.	Small amounts of mucoid stool, sometimes bloody	Colitis (see Glossary)	(C) See veterinarian for symptomatic treatment, dietary recommendations, or treatment for whipworms Also see Diarrhea
Straining to move bowels	Acute. Stool hard, contains foreign material (e.g., rocks, dirt, bone chips)	Possible vomiting	Foreign body in intestinal tract, causing constipation	(+) Will often take care of itself once the material passes. Could give stool softeners. Prevent dog from eating bones that can be chewed up or ingesting rocks/dirt. (24) If straining persists, see veterinarian

Sign/Symptom	Observations	Associated Signs	Possible Condition	Action to Take
Straining to move bowels	Progressive, chronic problem	Stools may be thinner than normal, but of normal consistency	Obstruction of colon or rectum due to: tumor; enlarged prostate; stricture or constriction from pelvic fracture	See veterinarian for rectal examination and possible X rays
Straining to move bowels	Usually unaltered male dog	Bulge to side of rectum	Perineal hernia	See veterinarian for rectal examination. Will probably require altering dog and surgically repairing the hernia.
Seems uncomfortable when moving bowels	Dog may be quiet, may lick rectum. May "scoot," or drag rectum on floor.	Red/purple swelling near rectum. Bloody discharge from opening in the swelling.	Anal sac abscess	Clean area if there is a discharge. Use warm compress to encourage drainage. See veterinarian. Will probably need to ensure proper drainage and give antibiotics.

Call veterinarian; make appointment immediately Life-threatening condition; go *immediately* to veterinarian or emergency clinic

Thirst, Changes in

If a dog drinks excessively, the water must be excreted in urine. Therefore, increases in thirst and urination go hand in hand. A dog that drinks a lot will have difficulty holding her urine and will need to go out more frequently. Conversely, if a dog is producing excess urine for a medical reason, she will need to drink more water, or she will become dehydrated. This is technically referred to as polyuria (increased urine) and polydipsia (increased thirst), or PU/PD.

Sign/Symptom	Observations	Associated Signs	Possible Condition	Action to Take
PU/PD	Losing weight	Increased appetite	Diabetes mellitus (see Glossary)	See veterinarian for blood tests. Bring urine sample.
PU/PD	Potbelly	Increased appetite. Hair loss.	Cushing's syndrome (see Glossary)	See veterinarian for blood tests. Bring urine sample.
PU/PD	None	None	Psychogenic water consumption, or diabetes insipidus (see Glossary)	See veterinarian for tests. Bring urine sample.
PU/PD	Possible loss of appetite. Possible weight loss.	Possible bad breath (if kidney disease); vomiting, lethargy	Liver disease or kidney disease (infection, failure); hypercalcemia (see Glossary)	See veterinarian for tests. Bring urine sample.
PU/PD	Unspayed female. Possibly lethargic.	Might have vaginal discharge	Pyometra (see p. 51; see also Box, p. 113)	See veterinarian for X rays, laboratory test, surgery
PU/PD	Appetite increased. Taking cortisone.	None	Reaction to cortisone	Call veterinarian to discuss dose of medication and alternatives

✚ Home care; first aid   🐾 Call veterinarian   🐾24 Call veterinarian; make appointment within 24 hours

Urination, Abnormal

Increase in normal volume of urination is covered in **Thirst, Changes in.** Here, we will discuss straining to urinate and abnormal urine or urinary patterns.

Sign/Symptom	Observations	Associated Signs	Possible Condition	Action to Take
Bloody urine	May have trouble holding urine	Urinates frequently, in small quantities	Bladder infection with or without bladder stones	See veterinarian for medication and possible X ray. Bring urine sample.
Straining to urinate. Usually male dog.	Will try to urinate frequently and may dribble small amounts. Stands with leg up for a long time.	Possibly lethargic. Possibly vomiting. Possible bloody urine.	Urinary tract obstruction. Males: bladder stones; tumors; urethral spasms; prostate disease. Females: tumors; rarely stones.	Go to emergency clinic for examination, X rays, possible surgery
Bloody urine	None	Bleeding anywhere else (mouth, nose, in stool)	Bleeding disorder, caused by: rat poison or drugs (see pp. 47–48; 55; see also Appendix A, pp. 157–58). DIC (see Glossary); immune-mediated disorder; trauma, hemolytic anemia.	See veterinarian for tests
Leaking urine (incontinent) when sleeping	Usually spayed female dog	May also lick vulva	Incontinence, usually a presumed estrogen deficiency. Rarely, bladder or spinal cord problem.	See veterinarian for medication. Bring urine sample.

 Call veterinarian; make appointment immediately

 Life-threatening condition; go *immediately* to veterinarian or emergency clinic

Sign/Symptom	Observations	Associated Signs	Possible Condition	Action to Take
Urinating in the house	May seem to have lost housebreaking	May also move bowels in house	If older dog, consider Abnormal Geriatric Behavior. If young dog, consider training (see "Housebreaking Problems," pp. 39–40)	➕ Retrain dog. Seek help of trainer or behaviorist if necessary.
Urinating in the house	Unaltered male dog. May be episodic or continual. Possibly small breed.	None	Marking behavior (see "Housebreaking Problems," pp. 39–40)	📞 Speak to veterinarian about neutering/ castration, which may decrease, but not necessarily eliminate, this behavior. Bring urine sample for evaluation.
Urine very dark, golden yellow, or orange	May be lethargic with decreased appetite	Possibly vomiting. Mucous membranes or eyes yellow.	Jaundice (see Glossary) from liver disease or hemolytic anemia (see Glossary)	➕📞 Go to emergency clinic for tests

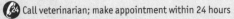

➕ Home care; first aid   📞 Call veterinarian   📞24 Call veterinarian; make appointment within 24 hours

Vomiting

Because of their tendency to "bolt" food and general lack of discrimination in what they will eat, dogs are apt to vomit more frequently than humans. Vomiting of undigested food usually takes place immediately after eating and, if it is not accompanied by signs of abdominal pain, diarrhea, or frequent retching, it should not be a cause for concern. Mild vomiting may be due to the ingestion of foreign material, a round-worm infestation (see page 16), or plant poisoning (see "Poisoning," pages 47–48; also see Appendix A, pages 157–58). If vomiting is accompanied by diarrhea, appetite loss, obvious distress or pain, distension of the abdomen, lethargy, or contains flecks or clots of blood, it can be a symptom of a systemic illness such as: canine distemper (see page 58); parvovirus ; diabetes mellitus (see Glossary); kidney failure, liver disease, pancreatitis, or a life-threatening emergency such as ruptured bowels, intestinal obstruction, or peritonitis. See Box, page 105, "Home Treatment of Routine Diarrhea or Vomiting."

Sign/Symptom	Observations	Associated Signs	Possible Condition	Action to Take
Acute, one to several times	Long, white, curled worms in vomitus	Possible diarrhea. Poor haircoat. Potbellied abdomen.	Roundworms, especially in puppies	See the veterinarian for medication. Take stool sample.
Acute, one to several times	Depression. Anorexia. Dehydration (see Box, p. 152).	Possible abdominal pain. Possible drooling. Possible diarrhea.	Intestinal obstruction. HGE (see Box, p. 102). Pancreatitis (see Glossary). Liver disease. Kidney disease. Severe intestinal parasites. Severe gastritis (see Glossary). Bacterial/ viral gastroenteritis. Addison's disease (see Glossary).	Go to veterinarian for examination, fluids, tests

 Call veterinarian; make appointment immediately

 Life-threatening condition; go *immediately* to veterinarian or emergency clinic

Sign/Symptom	Observations	Associated Signs	Possible Condition	Action to Take
Acute, one to several times	Anorexia. Depression. Abdominal Distension.	Drooling. Retching. Abdominal pain.	Gastric dilatation/ volvulus (GDV—see p. 50)	⊕ Go to emergency clinic for fluids, decompression, surgery
Acute, one to several times	Flecks or clots of blood in the vomitus	Possible black stool. Possible pale mucous membranes.	Gastric tumor. Gastric ulcer. Bleeding disorder. Gastric foreign body. Irritation from drugs.	🕐24 See the veterinarian for medication, X rays, tests
Acute, many times over a short period, or persistent	No response to fasting (see Box, "Home Treatment of Routine Diarrhea or Vomiting," p. 105), or vomiting recurs when food or water is offered	Dehydration. Depression/lethargy	Intestinal obstruction. Pancreatitis (see Glossary). Severe gastritis. Inflammatory bowel disease (IBD— see Glossary). Addison's disease (see Glossary). Liver disease. Kidney disease. Severe intestinal parasites. Stomach or intestinal tumor.	🕐 See the veterinarian for fluids, medication, tests, X rays

Dehydration in a Dog

A dog can become dehydrated because of loss of body fluids due to frequent or voluminous diarrhea or vomiting; a dog with heat prostration or one with a high fever will also become dehydrated, as will an animal deprived of drinking water. If a handful of a healthy dog's skin over the shoulders is lifted gently, it will bounce back in place immediately. When a dog is dehydrated his skin will lose its elasticity, become stiff, and fail to bounce back rapidly after it is lifted. (See illustration, p. 105).

⊕ Home care; first aid   🕐 Call veterinarian   🕐24 Call veterinarian; make appointment within 24 hours

Sign/Symptom	Observations	Associated Signs	Possible Condition	Action to Take
Chronic, several days or longer	Dog eats normally between bouts of vomiting; no weight loss	None	Food allergy. Chronic gastritis. Intestinal parasites. Dietary indiscretion.	Call the veterinarian for advice and medication. If you go to the office, bring stool sample.
Chronic, several days or longer	Weight loss	Possible anorexia. Possible dehydration. Possible depression. Possible diarrhea.	Inflammatory bowel disease (IBD—see Glossary). Addison's disease (see Glossary). Kidney disease. Liver disease. Gastrointestinal tumor. Intestinal obstruction. Pancreatitis. Severe intestinal parasites. Peritonitis (see Glossary).	See the veterinarian for tests, possible fluids, and X rays

Call veterinarian; make appointment immediately Life-threatening condition; go *immediately* to veterinarian or emergency clinic

153

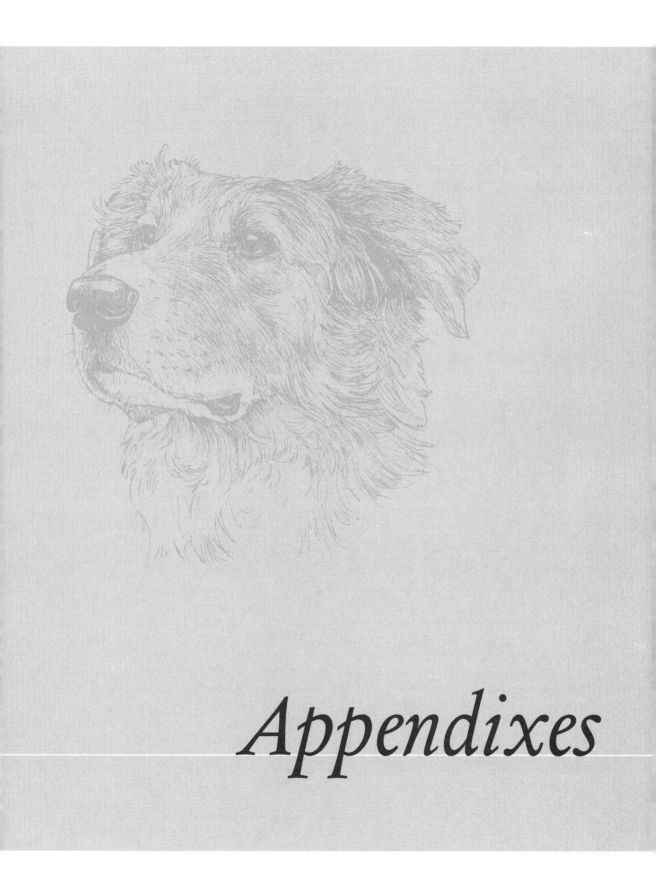

Appendixes

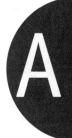

SOME COMMON HOUSEHOLD PRODUCTS THAT ARE POISONOUS

If a dog is known to have ingested any of these substances, take *immediately* to veterinarian or emergency clinic.

ASPCA National Animal Poison Control Center: 800-548-2423

Substance	Symptoms	Treatment
Antidepressant drugs	Vomiting, hyperexcitability, lack of balance, tremors, seizures, irregular heartbeat	Tranquilizers to counteract drug. Cardiac therapy.
Anti–flea and tick pesticides (collars, sprays, powders)	Vomiting, diarrhea, lack of balance	Fluid and drug therapy. Completely wash off any remaining drug.
Antifreeze	Mental confusion, vomiting, collapse, kidney failure, death	*Immediate veterinary treatment essential.* Intravenous fluid therapy. Activated charcoal. Specific antidotes.
Ammonium disinfectants (fabric softener)	Vomiting, diarrhea, neurological depression, seizures	*Dilute of milk/water. Activated charcoal. Saline cathartics. Supportive care for seizures, ulcers.
Aspirin and ibuprofen and other human pain relievers	Nausea, vomiting, stomach pain, possible lethargy	Intravenous fluids, sodium bicarbonate, other drugs
Bleaches	Salivation, vomiting due to ulceration	*Dilute of milk/water. Supportive care, gastrointestinal protectants.
Chocolate, caffeine	Vomiting, diarrhea, hyperactivity, possible seizures	*Emetics to induce vomiting, fluid therapy. Diazepam.

*May be given at home before *immediate* transportation to veterinarian or emergency clinic. Do not waste time. To induce vomiting, give one to two teaspoons of hydrogen peroxide (1:1, with water), or syrup of ipecac.

Substance	Symptoms	Treatment
Lead (paint, batteries, toys, shot, improperly glazed bowls)	Vomiting, abdominal distress, constipation or diarrhea, muscle spasms, hysteria, blindness	Blood test. Cathartics or surgery to remove lead. Corticosteroids. Systemic antidotes.
Onions, garlic	Anemia	Blood transfusion and fluids
Petroleum distillates (gasoline, fuels, solvents, paints)	Aspiration pneumonia if inhaled, burns if skin exposure	Oxygen. Rest. *If skin: wash with detergent or degreaser. If ingested: activated charcoal, gastric lavage. Supportive care.
Rodenticides		
Anticoagulant rat poison	Anemia, nosebleeds, gastrointestinal or urinary bleeding, bruising, difficulty breathing	Vitamin K injections. Blood transfusions. 2–4 weeks of therapy.
Cholecalciferol rat poison	Depression, vomiting, weakness	*Induce vomiting. Activated charcoal. Diuretics, fluids, other drugs.
Strychnine	Nervousness, stiffness, seizures	Activated charcoal. Sedation, gastric lavage. Diazepam or pentobarbital by IV. Fluid therapy.
Zinc phosphide	Severe gastritis, abdominal distension, vomiting, hypoglycemic shock, death	*Emetics. Absorbents. Rapid evacuation of stomach contents. Fluid therapy. Medications to reduce stomach acid.

*May be given at home before *immediate* transportation to veterinarian or emergency clinic. Do not waste time. To induce vomiting, give one to two teaspoons of hydrogen peroxide (1:1, with water), or syrup of ipecac.

SOME COMMON CONGENITAL DEFECTS AND DISORDERS*

(Note: This is *not* an exhaustive list. Most of these defects and disorders are extremely rare, and are only listed as possibilities.)

Breed/Color	Defects and/or Disorders
Afghan hound	*Afghan myelomalacia.* Softening of the tissues of the spinal cord, eventually causing paralysis. Usually occurs between 3 and 8 months of age.
	***Cataracts,* present at birth, may not be visible until 2 months of age and may be inherited. Juvenile cataracts may develop up to 6 years of age and heredity is the usual cause. In puppies, both types of cataracts may spontaneously disappear.
	Corneal dystrophy. Corneal dullness, usually in both eyes.
Airedale terrier	*Corneal dystrophy.* See "Afghan hound," directly above.
	Distichiasis. An extra row of eyelashes, which may rub on the cornea.
	IgA deficiency. Immune system deficiency, resulting in upper and lower respiratory infections, inflammation of the upper ear canal (otitis external), and skin problems.
	***Retinal dysplasia.* Abnormal development of the retina, which may lead to blindness.
	Triple-X syndrome. Females have 3 X chromosomes instead of 2, preventing normal cycling.
	Umbilical hernia. Swelling around the umbilicus (navel). May be surgically corrected.

Adapted, in part, from: *Textbook of Veterinary Internal Medicine,* Steven J. Ettinger, D.V.M., and Edward C. Feldman, D.V.M., editors. W. B. Saunders Co., Philadelphia. Appendix 2, "Congenital Defects of the Dog," Johnny D. Hoskins, D.V.M.

*Disorders are listed by specific breed. But also see "Large and Giant Breeds" and "Small and Toy Breeds."

**Prospective owners should screen parents and previous litters.

Breed/Color	Defects and/or Disorders
Akita—see also "Large and Giant Breeds"	*Deafness* in one or both ears.
	Microphthalmos. Failure of the eye globe to grow to normal size. May lead to blindness.
	Pseudo hyperkalemia. High level of potassium in red blood cells causing falsely elevated readings on clotted blood samples.
	***Retinal dysplasia.* Abnormal development of the retina, which may lead to blindness.
Alaskan malamute— see also "Large and Giant Breeds"	*Cartilaginous exostosis.* Outgrowths of cartilage from bones throughout the body.
	Chondrodysplasia. Dwarfism. Short front legs; paws turned sideways. Caused by poor cartilage and bone growth.
	Diabetes mellitus. May surface as early as 2–6 months of age. Characterized by high blood sugar, excessive thirst (polydipsia), and urination (polyuria).
	Factor VII deficiency. Lack of a blood-clotting-factor (prothrombin) blood plasma, often resulting in bleeding gums and nosebleeds.
	***Glaucoma.* Usually develops after 1 year of age. Caused by increase in eyeball pressure and can lead to blindness.
American Staffordshire terrier	*******Cataracts,* present at birth, may not be visible until 2 months of age and may be inherited. Juvenile cataracts may develop up to 6 years of age and heredity is the usual cause. In puppies, both types of cataracts may spontaneously disappear.
	Deafness in one or both ears.
	Myotonia. A disorder of the muscle fibers, resulting in difficulty relaxing muscles and causing a stiff gait.
Australian cattle dog/heeler	*******Cataracts,* present at birth, may not be visible until 2 months of age and may be inherited. Juvenile cataracts may develop up to 6 years of age and heredity is the usual cause. In puppies, both types of cataracts may spontaneously disappear.

**Prospective owners should screen parents and previous litters.

B

Breed/Color	Defects and/or Disorders
	Deafness in one or both ears.
Australian shepherd—see "Shepherds"	
Basenji	***Familial renal (kidney) disease,* which varies with individuals. May cause anorexia, lethargy, weight loss, anemia, excessive thirst (polydipsia) and urination (polyuria), and other problems.
	Fanconi's syndrome. Kidney tubule defects leading to the excessive loss of protein and other substances in the urine. Weight loss and kidney failure may result.
	Inguinal hernia. Hernia in the groin.
	***Optic nerve colobomas.* Pits or holes in the optic disc. Vision may be impaired.
	***Persistent pupillary membranes.* Membranes from the back of the eye attached to the backside of the cornea.
	Pyruvate kinase deficiency. An enzyme deficiency causing premature red blood cell destruction and anemia.
	Umbilical hernia. Swelling around the umbilicus (navel). May be surgically corrected.
Basset hound— see also "Large and Giant Breeds"	*Appendicular achondroplasia.* Cartilage at the ends of the long bones grows irregularly and is scant.
	Color mutant alopecia. Partial hair loss, dry coat, scaliness, and raised red spots on skin, combined with darkening of coat in patches.
	Combined immunodeficiency, causing severe bacterial skin, ear, respiratory, and intestinal infections beginning at birth.
	Cystinuria. A defect in the kidneys causing excessive cystine (an amino acid) in the urine, which leads to kidney and urinary tract stones.
	Ectropion. Eyelid turned outward, exposing mucous membranes covering the conjunctival lining, causing infection, ocular discharge, and swelling of the eyelid.
	***Glaucoma.* Caused by increased eyeball pressure and can lead to blindness. Usually develops after 1 year of age.

**Prospective owners should screen parents and previous litters.

Breed/Color	Defects and/or Disorders
Basset hound (cont'd)	*Inguinal hernia*. Hernia in the groin.
	Lysosomal storage diseases. Brain disorders caused by an inheritable deficiency of key enzymes.
	Thrombopathia. Blood-platelet disorder, causing nosebleeds, bleeding gums, and subcutaneous bruising.
Beagle	*Alopecia universalis*. A lack of hair cover all over the body.
	Brachury. An abnormally short tail.
	***Cataracts,* present at birth, may not be visible until 2 months of age and may be inherited. Juvenile cataracts may develop up to 6 years of age and heredity is the usual cause. In puppies, both types of cataracts may spontaneously disappear.
	Cleft palate/cleft lip syndrome. Midline closing defect affecting the lips and hard palate of the mouth.
	Cutaneous asthenia (Ehlers-Danlos syndrome). An abnormality of the connective tissue of the skin, resulting in loose, sagging skin that tears easily.
	Deafness in one or both ears.
	Epilepsy. Seizures, convulsions.
	Exocrine pancreatic insufficiency (EPI). Lack of pancreatic enzymes, resulting in poor digestion, excessive hunger, weight loss, and diarrhea.
	Factor VII deficiency. Lack of a blood-clotting-factor (prothrombin) blood plasma, often resulting in bleeding gums and nosebleeds.
	**Glaucoma. Usually develops after 1 year of age. Caused by increase in eyeball pressure and can lead to blindness.
	IgA deficiency. Immune system deficiency, resulting in upper and lower respiratory infections, inflammation of the upper ear canal (otitis external), and skin problems.
	Lysosomal storage diseases. Brain disorders caused by an inheritable deficiency of key enzymes.

**Prospective owners should screen parents and previous litters.

Breed/Color	Defects and/or Disorders
	Microphthalmos. Failure of the eye globe to grow to normal size. May lead to blindness.
	Narcolepsy-cataplexy. Excessive daytime sleep; muscle weakness, collapse.
	Nonspherocytic hemolytic anemia. Mild anemia caused by abnormal red blood cells.
	****Optic nerve hypoplasia.* Underdevelopment of the optic nerve in one or both eyes.
	Pulmonic stenosis. Narrowing or obstruction of artery leading from right ventricle of the heart to the pulmonary artery. May produce heart failure.
	Pyruvate kinase deficiency. An enzyme deficiency causing premature red blood destruction and anemia.
	****Retinal dysplasia.* Abnormal development of the retina, which may lead to blindness.
	Spina bifida. A defective fusion of spinal vertebrae causing paralysis.
	XX sex reversal, causing hermaphroditism and abnormal genital development.
Bedlington terrier	****Cataracts,* present at birth, may not be visible until 2 months of age and may be inherited. Juvenile cataracts may develop up to 6 years of age and heredity is the usual cause. In puppies, both types of cataracts may spontaneously disappear.
	Copper-associated hepatopathy. An overaccumulation of copper in the liver as dog ages, causing hepatitis and cirrhosis of the liver.
	Distichiasis. An extra row of eyelashes, which may rub on the cornea.
	Imperforate lacrimal punctum. Watering of the eye(s) due to improperly formed duct from the eye to the nose.
	Microphthalmos. Failure of the eye globe to grow to normal size. May lead to blindness.
	****Retinal dysplasia.* Abnormal development of the retina, which may lead to blindness.

**Prospective owners should screen parents and previous litters.

Breed/Color	Defects and/or Disorders
Belgian shepherd—see "Shepherds"	
Bernese mountain dog	*Hypomyelination/dysmyelination*. Reduced/abnormal insulating layer of myelin (material formed of protein and a lipid) around the central nervous system, causing rear limb weakness and difficulty walking.
Bichon Frise—see also "Small and Toy Breeds"	*Corneal dystrophy*. Corneal dullness, usually in both eyes.
	Primary ciliary dyskinesia. Abnormal functioning of small, hairlike processes in the respiratory system, leading to pneumonia.
Bloodhound	*Ectropion*. Eyelid turned outward, exposing mucous membranes covering the conjunctival lining, causing infection, ocular discharge, and swelling of the eyelid.
Border collie—see "Collies"	
Borzoi—see also "Large and Giant Breeds"	*Lymphedema*. Swelling and pitting of legs, usually hind legs, caused by abnormally developed lymph vessels.
	Methemoglobinemia. An enzyme deficiency, causing bluish to brownish mucous membranes, and dark, brownish blood that does not turn red when exposed to oxygen, resulting in fatigue, hypoxia, and death.
	Progressive retinal degeneration. Retinal lesions that first occur at 6 months of age, leading to blindness.
Boston terrier—see also "Brachycephalic Breeds"	**Cataracts,** present at birth, may not be visible until 2 months of age and may be inherited. Juvenile cataracts may develop up to 6 years of age and heredity is the usual cause. In puppies, both types of cataracts may spontaneously disappear.
	Cerebellar hypoplasia. Underdevelopment of the back part of the brain, characterized by lack of balance.
	Color mutant alopecia. Partial hair loss, dry coat, scaliness, and raised red spots on skin, combined with darkening of coat in patches.
	Deafness in one or both ears.

**Prospective owners should screen parents and previous litters.

Breed/Color	Defects and/or Disorders
	Diabetes insipidus. A metabolic disorder due to deficiency of a pituitary hormone, characterized by intense thirst (polydipsia) and large volumes of dilute urine (polyuria).
	Hydrocephalus. Accumulation of excess fluid in the brain and spinal cord, causing an enlarged head.
	Hypospadias. Abnormal location of male urinary orifice, often on the underside of the penis. May be corrected surgically.
	Ichthyosis. Dry, rough, thick, scaly skin, including footpads, which worsens with age.
	Pyloric stenosis. A narrowing of the muscular outlet of the stomach, causing frequent vomiting, distension of the stomach, weight loss, and cramping. May be corrected surgically.
Bouvier des Flandres—see also "Large and Giant Breeds"	*Glaucoma.* Usually develops after 1 year of age. Caused by an increase in eyeball pressure and can lead to blindness.
	Laryngeal paralysis. Paralysis of the larynx, resulting in loud, difficult breathing.
Boxer—see also "Brachycephalic Breeds"	***Aortic stenosis.* A narrowing of the opening of the aortic valve, which obstructs the flow of blood and can lead to fainting, collapse, and sudden death.
	Atrial anomalies. Defects of the upper chambers of the heart.
	Cryptorchidism. In which neither, or only one, testicle descends.
	Cutaneous asthenia (Ehlers-Danlos syndrome). An abnormality of the connective tissue of the skin, resulting in loose, sagging skin, which tears easily.
	Deafness in one or both ears, especially in white-coated dogs.
	Distichiasis. An extra row of eyelashes, which may rub on the cornea.
	Factor II deficiency. Lack of a blood-clotting factor, leading to mild bleeding, lameness, and nosebleeds. Trauma or surgery may lead to life-threatening bleeding.

**Prospective owners should screen parents and previous litters.

Breed/Color	Defects and/or Disorders
Boxer (cont'd)	*Factor VII deficiency.* Lack of a blood-clotting-factor (prothrombin) blood plasma, often resulting in bleeding gums or nosebleeds.
	Pyloric stenosis. A narrowing of the muscular outlet of the stomach, causing frequent vomiting, distension of the stomach, weight loss, and cramping. May be corrected surgically.
Brachycephalic Breeds—Affenpinscher, Boston terrier, boxer, Brussels griffon, bulldogs, Japanese chin, Lhasa apso, Pekingese, pug	*Cleft palate/cleft lip syndrome.* Midline closing defect affecting the lips and hard palate of the mouth.
	Corneal abrasion, due to protruding eyes and facial folds.
	Hiatal hernia. In which the stomach passes partially into the chest cavity through a hole in the esophagus.
	Prognathism. Upper jaw shorter than lower.
	Pyloric stenosis. A narrowing of the muscular outlet of the stomach, causing frequent vomiting, distension of the stomach, weight loss, and cramping. May be corrected surgically.
	Stenotic nares. An abnormal narrowing of the nasal passages, predisposing to loud, difficult mouth breathing, snoring, overheating, and other breathing difficulties.
	Tracheal collapse. Collapsed windpipe leading to coughing, bronchitis, and pneumonia.
	Tracheal hypoplasia. An underdeveloped windpipe, leading to pneumonia.
Brittany spaniel—see "Spaniels"	
Brussels griffon—see also "Brachycephalic Breeds" and "Small and Toy Breeds"	*Brachury.* An abnormally short tail.

Breed/Color	Defects and/or Disorders
	Shoulder luxation. Dislocation of the shoulder joint, occurring at 3–4 months of age.
Bulldogs—see also "Brachycephalic Breeds"	*Cystinuria*. A defect in the kidneys, causing excessive cystine (an amino acid) in the urine, which leads to kidney and urinary-tract stones.
	Factor VII deficiency. Lack of a blood-clotting-factor (prothrombin) blood plasma, often resulting in bleeding gums and nosebleeds.
English bulldog	*Anasarca*. Swelling of the legs, body, and genitals due to fluid retention.
	Brachury. Abnormally short tail.
	Cryptorchidism. In which neither, or only one, testicle descends.
	Deafness in one or both ears.
	Distichiasis. An extra row of eyelashes, which may rub on the cornea.
	Hydrocephalus. Accumulation of excess fluid in the brain and spinal cord, causing an enlarged head.
	Lymphedema. Swelling and pitting of the legs, usually hind legs, caused by abnormally developed lymph vessels.
	Mitral valve malformation. A malformation of the mitral valve in the left side of the heart, leading to heart murmur and eventual heart failure.
	Pulmonic stenosis. Narrowing or obstruction of artery leading from right ventricle of the heart to the pulmonary artery. May produce heart failure.
	Spina bifida. A defective fusion of spinal vertebrae causing paralysis.
	Ventricular septal defect. A hole in the wall (septum) between the left and right ventricles of the heart, producing a heart murmur and possible heart failure.
French bulldog	*Ununited anconeal process*. Elbow dysplasia. May occur in one or both front legs and may result in arthritis.
Bull terrier	*Cerebellar hypoplasia*. Underdevelopment of the back part of the brain, characterized by lack of balance.
	Deafness in one or both ears.

Breed/Color	Defects and/or Disorders
Bull terrier (cont'd)	*Ichthyosis.* Dry, rough, thick, scaly skin, including footpads, which worsens with age.
Cairn terrier	*Cryptorchidism,* in which neither, or only one, testicle descends.
	Hepatic cysts. Cysts on the liver that may lead to liver function problems.
	Hydrocephalus. Accumulation of excess fluid in the brain and spinal cord, causing an enlarged head.
	Inguinal hernia. Hernia in the groin.
	Lysosomal storage diseases. Brain disorders caused by an inheritable deficiency of key enzymes.
	Polycystic kidneys. A number of fluid-filled cysts on the kidneys that may result in kidney failure.
Cavalier King Charles spaniel—see "Spaniels"	
Chesapeake Bay retriever—see "Retrievers"	
Chihuahua—see also "Small and Toy Breeds"	*Atlantoaxial luxation.* Instability of cervical spine, which may lead to spinal injury.
	Color mutant alopecia. Partial hair loss, dry coat, scaliness, and raised red spots on skin, combined with darkening of coat in patches.
	Cryptorchidism, in which neither, or only one, testicle descends.
	Cystinuria. A defect in the kidneys, causing excessive cystine (an amino acid) in the urine, which leads to kidney and urinary-tract stones.
	Hydrocephalus. Accumulation of excess fluid in the brain and spinal cord, causing an enlarged head.
	Lysosomal storage diseases. Brain disorders caused by an inheritable deficiency of key enzymes.
	Mitral valve malformation. A malformation of the mitral valve of the left side of the heart, leading to heart murmur and eventual heart failure.
	Occipital dysplasia. Malformation of the occipital bone at the back and base of the skull, possibly exposing the cerebellum and brain stem to trauma.

Breed/Color	Defects and/or Disorders
	Persistent open fontanels. Soft spot in the center of the top of the skull, often associated with hydrocephalus.
	Primary ciliary dyskinesia. Abnormal functioning of small, hairlike processes in the respiratory system, leading to pneumonia.
	Pulmonic stenosis. Narrowing or obstruction of artery leading from the right ventricle of the heart to the pulmonary artery. May produce heart failure.
	Shoulder luxation. Dislocation of the shoulder joint, occurring at 3–4 months of age.
Chow chow	*Cerebellar hypoplasia.* Underdevelopment of the back part of the brain, characterized by lack of balance.
	Color mutant alopecia. Partial hair loss, dry coat, scaliness, and raised red spots on skin, combined with darkening of coat in patches.
	Diabetes mellitus. May surface as early as 2–6 months of age. Characterized by high blood sugar, excessive thirst (polydipsia) and urination (polyuria).
	**Familial renal (kidney) disease,* which varies with individuals. May cause anorexia, lethargy, weight loss, anemia, excessive thirst (polydipsia) and urination (polyuria), and other problems.
	Hypomyelination/dysmyelination. Reduced/abnormal insulating layer of myelin (material formed of protein and a lipid) around the central nervous system, causing rear limb weakness and difficulty walking.
	Myotonia. A disorder of the muscle fibers resulting in difficulty relaxing muscles and causing a stiff gait.
	Persistent pupillary membranes. Membranes from the back of the eye attached to the backside of the cornea.
	Primary ciliary dyskinesia. Abnormal functioning of small, hairlike processes in the respiratory system, leading to pneumonia.
	Tyrosinase deficiency. An enzyme deficiency causing changes in the color of the tongue and mucous membranes.
Cocker spaniel—see "Spaniels"	

**Prospective owners should screen parents and previous litters.

Breed/Color	Defects and/or Disorders
Collies	**Collie eye anomaly*. Multiple eye defects including coloboma of the optic disc.
	Deafness in one or both ears, particularly white-coated dogs.
	Dermatomyositis. Inflammation of skin and muscles, probably caused by an abnormal immune system.
	Epilepsy. Seizures, convulsions.
	Hypersensitivity to Ivermectin, a drug commonly used in prevention and treatment of heartworms.
	Microphthalmos. Failure of the eye globe to grow to normal size. May lead to blindness.
	***Optic nerve hypoplasia*. Underdevelopment of the optic nerve in one or both eyes.
	Patent ductus arteriosus. A condition in which a fetal blood vessel does not close at birth, causing a heart murmur and leading to heart failure.
	***Progressive retinal atrophy,* producing progressive vision loss, ending in blindness.
Border collie	*Lysosomal storage diseases*. Brain disorders caused by an inheritable deficiency of key enzymes.
	Primary ciliary dyskinesia. Abnormal functioning of small, hairlike processes in the respiratory system, leading to pneumonia.
	Selective cobalamin malabsorption. Erratic absorption of vitamin B12, causing anemia, weakness, and personality changes.
Grey collie	*Cyclic neutropenia*. Cyclic interruption in bone marrow production of white blood cells leading to infections and fever.
Corgis, Welsh Cardigan	***Progressive retinal atrophy*. An inheritable disorder, producing progressive vision loss, ending in blindness.
	***Retinal dysplasia*. Abnormal development of the retina, which may lead to blindness.
**Prospective owners should screen parents and previous litters.	

**Prospective owners should screen parents and previous litters.

Breed/Color	Defects and/or Disorders
Corgis, Pembroke	*Dermatomyositis.* Inflammation of skin and muscles, probably caused by an abnormal immune system.
	Renal telangiectasia. Blood loss in the urine from a serious kidney blood-vessel abnormality.
	***Retinal dysplasia*—see Cardigan, above.
Dachshund	*Appendicular achondroplasia.* Cartilage at the ends of the long bones grows irregularly and is scant.
	Cleft palate/cleft lip syndrome. Midline closing defect affecting the lips and hard palate of the mouth.
	Color mutant alopecia. Partial hair loss, dry coat, scaliness, and raised red spots on skin, combined with darkening of coat in patches.
	Cryptorchidism, in which neither, or only one, testicle descends.
	Cutaneous asthenia (Ehlers-Danlos syndrome). An abnormality of the connective tissue of the skin, resulting in loose, sagging skin, which tears easily.
	Cystinuria. A defect in the kidneys, causing excessive cystine (an amino acid) in the urine, which leads to kidney and urinary-tract stones.
	Deafness in one or both ears.
	Dermoid. A cyst on the eyelid. May affect one or both eyes.
	Enlargement of parotid salivary gland. Profuse drooling, caused by enlarged saliva glands.
	Epilepsy. Seizures, convulsions.
	Idiopathic megaesophagus. A disorder causing enlargement of the esophagus and leading to regurgitation of food and weight loss.
	Lysosomal storage diseases. Brain disorders caused by an inheritable deficiency of key enzymes.
	Microphthalmos. Failure of the eye globe to grow to normal size. May lead to blindness.

**Prospective owners should screen parents and previous litters.

Breed/Color	Defects and/or Disorders
Dachschund, cont'd	*Narcolepsy-cataplexy.* Excessive daytime sleep; muscle weakness, collapse.
	**Optic nerve hypoplasia.* Underdevelopment of the optic nerve in one or both eyes.
	Osteoporosis. Loss of bone tissue, causing weak bones. Puppies may be "swimmers," unable to stand.
	Portosystemic venous shunts. Abnormal blood vessel in the abdomen carries blood around, rather than through, the liver. Results in a buildup of toxins, which causes poor growth, salivation, seizures, and death. Surgery can help.
Dalmatian	*Deafness* in one or both ears.
	Dermoid. A cyst on the eyelid. May affect one or both eyes.
	Primary ciliary dyskinesia. Abnormal functioning of small, hairlike processes in the respiratory system, leading to pneumonia.
	Scotty cramp. Leg cramps caused by excitement or exercise. Usually begins at 6–8 weeks of age.
	Urate stone formation. Defect in uric acid transport, leads to production of urate kidney and urinary-tract stones.
Doberman pinscher—see "Pinschers"	
Elkhound—see "Norwegian elkhound"	
English bulldog—see "Bulldogs"	
English cocker spaniel—see "Spaniels"	
English pointer—see "Pointers"	
English setter—see "Setters"	
English sheepdog—see "Old English sheepdog"	
English springer spaniel—see "Spaniels"	
Finnish spitz	*Diabetes mellitus.* May surface as early as 2–6 months of age. Characterized by high blood sugar, excessive thirst (polydipsia) and urination (polyuria).

**Prospective owners should screen parents and previous litters.

Breed/Color	Defects and/or Disorders
	**Pituitary dwarfism*. Caused by a deficiency of growth hormone. Results in lack of permanent teeth, retention of puppy coat, abnormal skeletal growth, and many other disorders.
Foxhound	*Deafness* in one or both ears.
Fox terrier (smooth-coated and wirehaired)	***Ataxia of fox terriers*. Absence of myelin sheath (material formed of protein and a lipid) from the spinal cord, causing an unsteady gait.
	Cerebellar hypoplasia. Underdevelopment of the back part of the brain, characterized by lack of balance.
	Cervical vertebral instability. Malformation of the spinal cord, resulting in an inability to walk properly—"wobbler syndrome."
	Deafness in one or both ears.
	Ectopic ureter. A misplacement of the tube or tubes that lead from the kidneys to the bladder. Females, especially, are often incontinent.
	***Glaucoma*. Usually develops after 1 year of age. Caused by an increase in eyeball pressure and can lead to blindness.
	Legg-Calvé-Perthes disease (aseptic necrosis). Collapse of bone and malformation of the hip joint, leading to arthritis. Onset at 5–9 months of age. May be corrected surgically.
	Myasthenia gravis. A disease that may surface at 6–9 weeks of age or older. It causes muscle weakness, including an inability to blink both eyes, breathing difficulty, and regurgitation.
	Pulmonic stenosis. Narrowing or obstruction of artery leading from right ventricle of the heart to the pulmonary artery. May produce heart failure.
	Shoulder luxation. Dislocation of the shoulder joint, occurring at 3–4 months of age.
French bulldog—see "Bulldogs"	
German shepherd—see "Shepherds"	
German shorthaired pointer—see "Pointers"	
**Prospective owners should screen parents and previous litters.	

SOME COMMON CONGENITAL DEFECTS AND DISORDERS

Breed/Color	Defects and/or Disorders
Giant breeds—see "Large and Giant Breeds"	
Giant schnauzer—see "Schnauzers"	
Golden retriever—see "Retrievers"	
Gordon setter—see "Setters"	
Great Dane—see also "Large and Giant Breeds"	*Color mutant alopecia.* Partial hair loss, dry coat, scaliness, and raised red spots on skin, combined with darkening of coat in patches.
	Deafness in one or both ears.
	Enophthalmos. A sinking of the eyeball into the socket.
	Idiopathic megaesophagus. A disorder causing enlargement of the esophagus and leading to regurgitation of food and weight loss.
	Lymphedema. Swelling and pitting of the legs, usually hind legs, caused by abnormally developed lymph vessels.
	Microphthalmos. Failure of the eye globe to grow to normal size. May lead to blindness.
	Mitral valve malformation. A malformation of the mitral valve in the left side of the heart, leading to a heart murmur and eventual heart failure.
	Myotonia. A disorder of the muscle fibers, resulting in difficulty relaxing muscles and causing a stiff gait.
	Tricuspid valve dysplasia. A malformation of the tricuspid valve of the right side of the heart. Leads to heart murmur and heart failure.
Great Pyrenees—see also "Large and Giant Breeds"	*Deafness* in one or both ears.
	Factor XI deficiency. A deficiency of a clotting factor in the blood, causing minor bleeding. Trauma or surgery may produce major bleeding.
	***Optic nerve hypoplasia.* Underdevelopment of the optic nerve in one or both eyes.

**Prospective owners should screen parents and previous litters.

Breed/Color	Defects and/or Disorders
Greyhound	*Color mutant alopecia.* Partial hair loss, dry coat, scaliness, and raised red spots on skin, combined with darkening of coat in patches.
	Cutaneous asthenia (Ehlers-Danlos syndrome). An abnormality of the connective tissue of the skin, resulting in loose, sagging skin, which tears easily.
Ibizan hound	*Deafness* in one or both ears.
Irish setter—see "Setters"	
Irish terrier	*Cystinuria.* A defect in the kidneys causing excessive cystine (an amino acid) in the urine, which leads to kidney and urinary-tract stones.
	Digital hyperkeratosis. Thickening of the footpads, making them split easily, become infected and painful.
	X-linked muscular dystrophy. Causes a stiff gait ("bunny hop"). Appears at 6–9 weeks of age.
Irish wolfhound—see also "Large and Giant Breeds"	*Portosystemic venous shunts.* Abnormal blood vessel in the abdomen carries blood around, rather than through, the liver. Results in a buildup of toxins, which causes poor growth, salivation, seizures, and death. Surgery can help.
Jack Russell terrier—see also "Small and Toy Breeds"	******Ataxia of fox terriers.* Absence of myelin sheath from the spinal cord, causing an unsteady gait.
	Myasthenia gravis. A disease that may surface at 6–9 weeks of age or older. It causes muscle weakness, including an inability to blink both eyes, breathing difficulty, and regurgitation.
Japanese mongrel	*Pseudo hyperkalemia.* High level of potassium in red blood cells causing falsely elevated readings on clotted blood samples.
Keeshond	*Diabetes mellitus.* May surface as early as 2–6 months of age. Characterized by high blood sugar, excessive thirst (polydipsia), and urination (polyuria).
	Epilepsy. Seizures, convulsions.
	Patent ductus arteriosus. A condition in which a fetal blood vessel does not close at birth, causing a heart murmur and leading to heart failure.

**Prospective owners should screen parents and previous litters.

Breed/Color	Defects and/or Disorders
Keeshond (cont'd)	*Tetralogy of Fallot.* A very serious combination of four heart defects leading to poor oxygenation and early death.
	Ventricular septal defect. A hole in the wall (septum) between the left and right ventricles of the heart, producing a heart murmur and possible heart failure.
Kerry blue terrier	*Cerebellar abiotrophy.* Serious disorder of the brain.
	Factor X deficiency. A deficiency of a clotting factor in the blood, causing minor bleeding. Trauma or surgery may produce major bleeding.
	XX sex reversal, causing hermaphroditism and abnormal genital development.
Kuvasz	*Deafness* in one or both ears.
Labrador retriever—see "Retrievers"	
Large and Giant Breeds— Akita; Alaskan malamute; basset hound; borzoi; Bouvier des Flandres; Great Dane; Great Pyrenees; Irish wolfhound; Newfoundland; Old English sheepdog; retrievers; Russian wolfhound; schnauzer, giant; Scottish deerhound; shepherds	*Cervical vertebral instability.* Malformation of the spinal cord, resulting in an inability to walk properly—"wobbler syndrome."
	***Hip dysplasia.* A deformity of the hip joint, leading to lameness. Onset usually occurs at about 5 months of age.
	Panosteitis. Lameness due to rapid growth and inflammation of long bones.
	Ununited anconeal process. Elbow dysplasia. May occur in one or both front legs and may result in arthritis.

**Prospective owners should screen parents and previous litters.

Breed/Color	Defects and/or Disorders
	Vaginal prolapse—females. A downward displacement of the vagina causing it to protrude outside the body.
Lhasa apso—see also "Brachycephalic Breeds" and "Small and Toy Breeds"	****Familial renal (kidney) disease,* which varies with individuals. May cause anorexia, lethargy, weight loss, anemia, excessive thirst (polydipsia) and urination (polyuria), and other problems.
	Hydrocephalus. Accumulation of excess fluid in the brain and spinal cord, causing an enlarged head.
Lundehund	*Intestinal lymphangiectasia.* Leakage of blood protein into intestinal tract through abnormal lymphatic vessels, leading to edema and hypoproteinemia.
Maltese—see also "Small and Toy Breeds"	*Cryptorchidism,* in which neither, or only one, testicle descends.
	Deafness in one or both ears.
	Hydrocephalus. Accumulation of excess fluid in the brain and spinal cord, causing an enlarged head.
Manchester terrier	*Diabetes mellitus.* May surface as early as 2–6 months of age. Characterized by high blood sugar, excessive thirst (polydipsia), and urination (polyuria).
	Legg-Calvé-Perthes disease (aseptic necrosis). Collapse of bone and malformation of the hip joint, leading to arthritis. Onset at 5–9 months of age. May be corrected surgically.
Miniature breeds—see "Small and Toy Breeds"	
Newfoundland—see also "Large and Giant Breeds"	****Aortic stenosis.* A narrowing of the opening of the aortic valve, which obstructs the flow of blood and can lead to fainting, collapse, and sudden death.
	Cystinuria. A defect in the kidneys causing excessive cystine (an amino acid) in the urine, which leads to kidney and urinary-tract stones.
Norwegian elkhound	*Diabetes insipidus.* A metabolic disorder due to deficiency of a pituitary hormone, characterized by intense thirst (polydipsia) and large volumes of dilute urine (polyuria).

**Prospective owners should screen parents and previous litters.

Breed/Color	Defects and/or Disorders
Norwegian elkhound (cont'd)	*Diabetes mellitus.* May surface as early as 2–6 months of age. Characterized by high blood sugar, excessive thirst (polydipsia) and urination (polyuria).
	***Familial renal (kidney) disease,* which varies with individuals. May cause anorexia, lethargy, weight loss, anemia, excessive thirst (polydipsia) and urination (polyuria), and other problems.
	***Progressive retinal atrophy,* producing progressive vision loss, ending in blindness.
Old English sheepdog—see also "Large and Giant Breeds"	*Atrial anomalies.* Defects of the upper chambers of the heart.
	***Cataracts,* present at birth, may not be visible until 2 months of age and may be inherited. Juvenile cataracts may develop up to 6 years of age and heredity is the usual cause. In puppies, both types of cataracts may spontaneously disappear.
	Deafness in one or both ears.
	Diabetes mellitus. May surface as early as 2–6 months of age. Characterized by high blood sugar, excessive thirst (polydipsia) and urination (polyuria).
	Lymphedema. Swelling and pitting of the legs, usually hind legs, caused by abnormally developed lymph vessels.
	Microphthalmos. Failure of the eye globe to grow to normal size. May lead to blindness.
	Primary ciliary dyskinesia. Abnormal functioning of small, hairlike processes in the respiratory system, leading to pneumonia.
	***Retinal dysplasia.* Abnormal development of the retina, which may lead to blindness.
	XX/XY chimeras with testes. Males have no external testes or scrotum.
Otterhound	*Thrombasthenic thrombopathia.* Defective blood platelets, retarding normal clotting.
Papillon—see also "Small and Toy Breeds"	*Deafness* in one or both ears.

**Prospective owners should screen parents and previous litters.

Breed/Color	Defects and/or Disorders
Pekingese—see also "Brachycephalic Breeds" and "Small and Toy Breeds"	*Atlantoaxial luxation.* Instability of cervical spine, which may lead to spinal injury.
	Cryptorchidism. In which neither, or only one, testicle descends.
	Distichiasis. An extra row of eyelashes, which may rub on the cornea.
	Hydrocephalus. Accumulation of excess fluid in the brain and spinal cord, causing an enlarged head.
	Inguinal hernia. Hernia in the groin.
	Legg-Calvé-Perthes disease (aseptic necrosis). Collapse of bone and malformation of the hip joint, leading to arthritis. Onset at 5–9 months of age. May be corrected surgically.
	Pseudohermaphroditism. Occurs in both females and males. The external genitalia do not match actual gender.
	Umbilical hernia. Swelling around the umbilicus (navel). May be surgically corrected.
Pinschers, Doberman	*Cervical vertebral instability.* Malformation of the spinal cord, resulting in an inability to walk properly—"wobbler syndrome."
	Color mutant alopecia. Partial hair loss, dry coat, scaliness, and raised red spots on skin, combined with darkening of coat in patches. Primarily affects blue-colored dogs.
	Copper-associated hepatopathy. An overaccumulation of copper in the liver as dog ages, causing hepatitis and cirrhosis of the liver.
	Deafness in one or both ears.
	Diabetes mellitus. May surface as early as 2–6 months of age. Characterized by high blood sugar, excessive thirst (polydipsia) and urination (polyuria).
	Enophthalmos. A sinking of the eyeball into the socket.
	Exocrine pancreatic insufficiency (EPI). Lack of pancreatic enzymes resulting in poor digestion, excessive hunger, weight loss, and diarrhea.

Breed/Color	Defects and/or Disorders
Pinschers, Doberman (cont'd)	******_Familial renal (kidney) disease,_ which varies with individuals. May cause anorexia, lethargy, weight loss, anemia, excessive thirst (polydipsia) and urination (polyuria), and other problems.
	Granulocytopathy. A defect in the body's ability to kill bacteria, causing stunted growth and recurring bacterial infections.
	Ichthyosis. Dry, rough, thick, scaly skin, including footpads, which worsens with age.
	Malposition of urinary bladder (pelvic bladder). May cause urinary incontinence.
	Microphthalmos. Failure of the eye globe to grow to normal size. May lead to blindness.
	Narcolepsy-cataplexy. Excessive daytime sleep; muscle weakness, collapse.
	Peripheral vestibular disorders, causing head tilt, circling, and rolling at birth or shortly thereafter.
	Portosystemic venous shunts. Abnormal blood vessel in the abdomen carries blood around, rather than through, the liver. Results in a buildup of toxins, which cause poor growth, salivation, seizures, and death. Surgery can help.
	Primary ciliary dyskinesia. Abnormal functioning of small, hairlike processes in the respiratory system, leading to pneumonia.
	**_Retinal dysplasia._ Abnormal development of the retina, which may lead to blindness.
	**_von Willebrand's disease, Factor VIII deficiency._ An inherited bleeding disorder.
	XO syndrome. Females do not cycle.
Pinschers, Miniature	_Mucopolysaccharidosis VI._ Decreased long-bone growth; corneal opacity.
	**_Pituitary dwarfism._ Caused by a deficiency of growth hormone. Results in lack of permanent teeth, retention of puppy coat, abnormal skeletal growth, and many other disorders.
Pointers	_Deafness_ in one or both ears.
	Motor neuronopathies. Defects in the nerves that control leg movement.

**Prospective owners should screen parents and previous litters.

Breed/Color	Defects and/or Disorders
English pointer	*Primary ciliary dyskinesia.* Abnormal functioning of small, hairlike processes in the respiratory system, leading to pneumonia.
German shorthaired pointer	*Aortic stenosis.* A narrowing of the opening of the aortic valve, which obstructs the flow of blood and can lead to fainting, collapse, and sudden death.
	Diabetes insipidus. A metabolic disorder due to a deficiency of a pituitary hormone, characterized by intense thirst (polydipsia) and large volumes of dilute urine (polyuria).
	Factor XII deficiency. A blood-clotting disorder not usually associated with bleeding.
	Lysosomal storage diseases. Brain disorders caused by an inheritable deficiency of key enzymes.
	XX sex reversal, causing hermaphroditism and abnormal genital development.
Pomeranian—see also "Brachycephalic breeds" and "Small and Toy Breeds"	*Atlantoaxial luxation.* Instability of cervical spine, which may lead to spinal injury.
	Cryptorchidism, in which neither, or only one, testicle descends.
	Hydrocephalus. Accumulation of excess fluid in the brain and spinal cord, resulting in an enlarged head.
	Lysosomal storage diseases. Brain disorders caused by an inheritable deficiency of key enzymes.
	Patent ductus arteriosus. A condition in which a fetal blood vessel does not close at birth, causing a heart murmur and leading to heart failure.
	Shoulder luxation. Dislocation of the shoulder joint, occurring at 3–4 months of age.
	Tracheal collapse. Collapsed windpipe, leading to coughing, bronchitis, and pneumonia.
Poodle, all sizes	*Appendicular achondroplasia.* Cartilage at the ends of the long bones grows irregularly and is scant.

Breed/Color	Defects and/or Disorders
Poodle, all sizes (cont'd)	*Atlantoaxial luxation.* Instability of cervical spine, which may lead to spinal injury.
	***Cataracts,* present at birth, may not be visible until 2 months of age and may be inherited. Juvenile cataracts may develop up to 6 years of age and heredity is the usual cause. In puppies, both types of cataracts may spontaneously disappear.
	Color mutant alopecia. Partial hair loss, dry coat, scaliness, and raised red spots on skin, combined with darkening of coat in patches.
	Cryptorchidism, in which neither, or only one, testicle descends.
	Deafness in one or both ears.
	Diabetes insipidus. A metabolic disorder due to a deficiency of a pituitary hormone, characterized by intense thirst (polydipsia) and large volumes of dilute urine (polyuria).
	Diabetes mellitus. May surface as early as 2–6 months of age. Characterized by high blood sugar, excessive thirst (polydipsia) and urination (polyuria).
	Distichiasis. An extra row of eyelashes, which may rub on the cornea.
	Ectopic ureter. A misplacement of the tube or tubes that lead from the kidneys to the bladder. Females, especially, are often incontinent.
	Factor XII deficiency. A blood-clotting disorder usually not associated with bleeding.
	***Familial renal (kidney) disease,* which varies with individuals. May cause anorexia, lethargy, weight loss, anemia, excessive thirst (polydipsia) and urination (polyuria), and other problems.
	***Glaucoma.* Usually develops after 1 year of age. Caused by increase in eyeball pressure and can lead to blindness.
	Hydrocephalus. Accumulation of excess fluid in the brain and spinal cord, causing an enlarged head.
	Legg-Calvé-Perthes disease (aseptic necrosis). Collapse of bone and malformation of the hip joint, leading to arthritis. Onset at 5–9 months of age. May be corrected surgically.

**Prospective owners should screen parents and previous litters.

Breed/Color	Defects and/or Disorders
	Lymphedema. Swelling and pitting of legs, usually hind legs, caused by abnormally developed lymph vessels.
	Lysosomal storage diseases. Brain disorders caused by an inheritable deficiency of key enzymes.
	Narcolepsy-cataplexy. Excessive daytime sleep; muscle weakness, collapse.
	***Optic nerve hypoplasia*. Underdevelopment of the optic nerve in one or both eyes.
	Patent ductus arteriosus. A condition in which a fetal blood vessel does not close at birth, causing a heart murmur and leading to heart failure.
	Portosystemic venous shunts. Abnormal blood vessel in the abdomen carries blood around, rather than through, the liver. Results in a buildup of toxins, which cause poor growth, salivation, seizures, and death. Surgery may help.
	Pseudohermaphroditism—males. In which the external genitalia do not match the actual gender.
	Pyruvate kinase deficiency. An enzyme deficiency causing premature red blood cell destruction and anemia.
	Shoulder luxation. Dislocation of the shoulder joint, occurring at 3–4 months of age.
	Tetralogy of Fallot. A very serious combination of four heart defects leading to poor oxygenation and early death.
	Tracheal collapse. Collapsed windpipe leading to coughing, bronchitis, and pneumonia.
Portuguese water dog	*Lysosomal storage diseases*. Brain disorders caused by an inheritable deficiency of key enzymes.
	Microphthalmos. Failure of the eye globe to grow to normal size. May lead to blindness.
Pug—see also "Brachycephalic Breeds"	*Distichiasis*. An extra row of eyelashes, which may rub on the cornea.

**Prospective owners should screen parents and previous litters.

Breed/Color	Defects and/or Disorders
Pug (cont'd)	*Hydrocephalus.* An accumulation of excess fluid in the brain and spinal cord, causing an enlarged head.
	Legg-Calvé-Perthes disease (aseptic necrosis). Collapse of bone and malformation of the hip joint, leading to arthritis. Onset at 5–9 months of age. May be corrected surgically.
	Pug encephalitis. An inflammation of the brain, causing seizures, circling, and personality changes.
	XX sex reversal, causing hermaphroditism and abnormal genital development.
Retrievers—see also "Large and Giant Breeds"	*Epilepsy.* Seizures, convulsions.
Chesapeake Bay retriever	*******Cataracts,* present at birth, may not be visible until 2 months of age and may be inherited. Juvenile cataracts may develop up to 6 years of age and heredity is the usual cause. In puppies, both types of cataracts may spontaneously disappear.
	***Retinal dysplasia.* Abnormal development of the retina, which may lead to blindness.
Golden retriever	*******Aortic stenosis.* A narrowing of the opening of the aortic valve, which obstructs the flow of blood and can lead to fainting, collapse, and sudden death.
	**Cataracts—see "Chesapeake Bay retriever," above.
	Diabetes mellitus. May surface as early as 2–6 months of age. Characterized by high blood sugar, excessive thirst (polydipsia) and urination (polyuria).
	Enophthalmos. A sinking of the eyeball into the socket.
	Hypomyelination/dysmyelination. Reduced/abnormal insulating layer of myelin (material formed of protein and a lipid) around the central nervous system, causing rear limb weakness and difficulty walking.
	Portosystemic venous shunts. Abnormal blood vessel in the abdomen carries blood around, rather than through, the liver. Results in a buildup of toxins, which cause poor growth, salivation, seizures, and death. Surgery can help.
	Primary ciliary dyskinesia. Abnormal functioning of small, hairlike processes in the respiratory system, leading to pneumonia.

**Prospective owners should screen parents and previous litters.

Breed/Color	Defects and/or Disorders
	von Willebrand's disease. Factor VIII deficiency. An inherited bleeding disorder.
	X-linked muscular dystrophy. Causes a stiff gait ("bunny hop"). Appears at 6–9 weeks of age.
Labrador retriever	*Chondrodysplasia.* Dwarfism. Short front legs; paws turned sideways. Caused by poor cartilage and bone growth.
	Cleft palate/cleft lip syndrome. Midline closing defect affecting the lips and hard palate of the mouth.
	Diabetes mellitus. May surface as early as 2–6 months of age. Characterized by high blood sugar, excessive thirst (polydipsia) and urination (polyuria).
	Ectopic ureter. Misplacement of the tube or tubes that lead from the kidneys to the bladder. Females, especially, are often incontinent.
	Exocrine pancreatic insufficiency (EPI). Lack of pancreatic enzymes resulting in poor digestion, excessive hunger, weight loss, and diarrhea.
	Familial myoclonus. Marked muscular hypertonicity (muscles that overcontract). Begins at 3 weeks of age.
	Labrador retriever myopathy. Progressive, degenerative muscle disease, causing a stiff gait ("bunny hop"). Begins at 3–4 months.
	Lymphedema. Swelling and pitting of the legs, usually hind legs, caused by abnormally developed lymph vessels.
	Microphthalmos. Failure of the eye globe to grow to normal size. May lead to blindness.
	Narcolepsy-cataplexy. Excessive daytime sleep; muscle weakness, collapse.
	Portosystemic venous shunts. Abnormal blood vessel in the abdomen carries blood around, rather than through, the liver. Results in a buildup of toxins, which causes poor growth, salivation, seizures, and death. Surgery can help.
	***Progressive retinal atrophy,** an inheritable disorder producing progressive vision loss, ending in blindness.

**Prospective owners should screen parents and previous litters.

Breed/Color	Defects and/or Disorders
Labrador retriever (cont'd)	******Retinal dysplasia. Abnormal development of the retina, which may lead to blindness.
Rhodesian ridgeback	Deafness in one or both ears.
	Myotonia. A disorder of the muscle fibers, resulting in difficulty relaxing muscles and causing a stiff gait.
Rottweiler—see also "Large and Giant Breeds"	Deafness in one or both ears.
	Motor neuronopathies. Disorders affecting motor neurons to muscles in limbs.
	**Retinal dysplasia. Abnormal development of the retina, which may lead to blindness.
	**von Willebrand's disease. Factor VIII deficiency. An inherited bleeding disorder.
	X-linked muscular dystrophy. Causes a stiff gait ("bunny hop"). Appears at 6–9 weeks of age.
Russian wolfhound—see also "Large and Giant Breeds"	Factor I deficiency. Deficiency of a blood-clotting factor, which may cause bleeding.
	**Optic nerve hypoplasia. Underdevelopment of the optic nerve in one or both eyes.
Saint Bernard (St. Bernard)—see also "Large and Giant Breeds"	Aphakia. Congenital absence of eye lens.
	Cervical vertebral instability. Malformation of the spinal cord, resulting in an inability to walk properly—"wobbler syndrome."
	Cutaneous asthenia (Ehlers-Danlos syndrome). An abnormality of the connective tissue of the skin, resulting in loose, sagging skin, which tears easily.
	Deafness in one or both ears.
	Distichiasis. An extra row of eyelashes, which may rub on the cornea.

**Prospective owners should screen parents and previous litters.

Breed/Color	Defects and/or Disorders
	Ectropion. Eyelid turned outward, exposing mucous membranes covering the conjunctival lining, causing infection, ocular discharge, and swelling of the eyelid.
	Enophthalmos. A sinking of the eyeball into the socket.
	Exocrine pancreatic insufficiency (EPI). Lack of pancreatic enzymes, resulting in poor digestion, excessive hunger, weight loss, and diarrhea.
	Factor I deficiency. Deficiency of a blood-clotting factor, which may cause bleeding.
	Narcolepsy-cataplexy. Excessive daytime sleep; muscle weakness, collapse.
	***Optic nerve hypoplasia.* Underdevelopment of the optic nerve in one or both eyes.
Saluki	*Lysosomal storage diseases.* Brain disorders caused by an inheritable deficiency of key enzymes.
Samoyed	*Atrial anomalies.* Defects of the upper chambers of the heart.
	***Familial renal (kidney) disease,* which varies with individuals. May cause anorexia, lethargy, weight loss, anemia, excessive thirst (polydipsia) and urination (polyuria), and other problems
	Glaucoma. Caused by increased eyeball pressure and can lead to blindness. Usually develops after 1 year of age.
	Hypomyelination/dysmyelination. Reduced/abnormal insulating layer of myelin (material formed of protein and a lipid) around the central nervous system, causing rear limb weakness and difficulty walking.
	Portosystemic venous shunts. Abnormal blood vessel in the abdomen carries blood around, rather than through, the liver. Results in a buildup of toxins, which causes poor growth, salivation, seizures, and death. Surgery can help.
	Pulmonic stenosis. Narrowing or obstruction of artery leading from right ventricle of the heart to the pulmonary artery. May produce heart failure.
	***Retinal dysplasia.* Abnormal development of the retina, which may lead to blindness.

**Prospective owners should screen parents and previous litters.

S O M E   C O M M O N   C O N G E N I T A L   D E F E C T S   A N D   D I S O R D E R S

Breed/Color	Defects and/or Disorders
Samoyed (cont'd)	*X-linked muscular dystrophy.* Causes a stiff gait ("bunny hop"). Appears at 6–9 weeks of age.
Schipperke	*Diabetes mellitus.* May surface as early as 2–6 months of age. Characterized by high blood sugar, excessive thirst (polydipsia) and urination (polyuria).
Schnauzers	*Cleft palate/cleft lip syndrome.* Midline closing defect affecting the lips and hard palate of the mouth.
	Diabetes insipidus. A metabolic disorder due to deficiency of a pituitary hormone, characterized by intense thirst (polydipsia) and large volumes of dilute urine (polyuria).
	Legg-Calvé-Perthes disease (aseptic necrosis). Collapse of bone and malformation of the hip joint, leading to arthritis. Onset at 5–9 months of age. May be corrected surgically.
	Tetralogy of Fallot. A very serious combination of four heart defects leading to poor oxygenation and early death.
Giant schnauzer—see also "Large and Giant Breeds"	*Hypothyroidism.* A subnormal activity of the thyroid gland, leading to lethargy, and skin and haircoat problems.
	***Pituitary dwarfism.* Caused by a deficiency of a growth hormone. Results in lack of permanent teeth, retention of puppy coat, abnormal skeletal growth, and many other disorders.
	Selective cobalamin malabsorption. Erratic absorption of vitamin B12, causing anemia, weakness, and personality changes.
Miniature schnauzer—see also "Small and Toy Breeds"	***Cataracts,* present at birth, may not be visible until 2 months of age and may be inherited. Juvenile cataracts may develop up to 6 years of age and heredity is the usual cause. In puppies, both types of cataracts may spontaneously disappear.
	Cryptorchidism, in which neither, or only one, testicle descends.
	Diabetes mellitus. May surface as early as 2–6 months of age. Characterized by high blood sugar, excessive thirst (polydipsia) and urination (polyuria).

**Prospective owners should screen parents and previous litters.

B

Breed/Color	Defects and/or Disorders
	Dysbetalipoproteinapathy. Defective fat metabolism leading to hyperlipidemia (abnormal fat in the blood), causing pancreatitis.
	Factor VII deficiency. Lack of a blood-clotting-factor (prothrombin) blood plasma, often resulting in bleeding gums and nosebleeds.
	Idiopathic megaesophagus. A disorder causing enlargement of the esophagus and leading to regurgitation of food and weight loss.
	Microphthalmos. Failure of the eye globe to grow to normal size. May lead to blindness.
	**Progressive retinal atrophy.* An inherited disorder producing progressive vision loss, ending in blindness.
	Pseudohermaphroditism—males. In which the external genitalia do not match the actual gender.
	Pulmonic stenosis. Narrowing or obstruction of artery leading from right ventricle of the heart to the pulmonary artery. May produce heart failure.
Standard schnauzer	**Retinal dysplasia.* Abnormal development of the retina, which may lead to blindness.
Scottish deerhound—see also "Large and Giant Breeds"	*Hypothyroidism.* A subnormal activity of the thyroid gland, leading to lethargy, and skin and haircoat problems.
Scottish terrier	*Appendicular achondroplasia.* Cartilage at the ends of the long bones grows irregularly and is scant.
	Deafness in one or both ears.
	Scotty cramp. Leg cramps caused by excitement or exercise. Usually begins at 6–8 weeks of age.
	***von Willebrand's disease. Factor VIII deficiency.* An inherited bleeding disorder.
Sealyham terrier	***Cataracts,* present at birth, may not be visible until 2 months of age and may be inherited. Juvenile cataracts may develop up to 6 months of age and heredity is the usual cause. In puppies, both types of cataracts may spontaneously disappear.

**Prospective owners should screen parents and previous litters.

Breed/Color	Defects and/or Disorders
Sealyham terrier (cont'd)	*Deafness* in one or both ears.
	Microphthalmos. Failure of the eye globe to grow to normal size. May lead to blindness.
	***Retinal dysplasia.* Abnormal development of the retina, which may lead to blindness.
Setters	*Epilepsy.* Seizures, convulsions.
English setter	*Deafness* in one or both ears.
	Lysosomal storage diseases. Brain disorders caused by an inheritable deficiency of key enzymes.
	Methemoglobinemia. An enzyme deficiency, causing bluish to brownish mucous membranes and dark, brownish blood that does not turn red when exposed to oxygen, resulting in fatigue, hypoxia, and death.
Gordon setter	*Cerebellar abiotrophies.* Serious disorder of the brain.
Irish setter	*Cerebellar hypoplasia.* Underdevelopment of the back part of the brain, characterized by lack of balance.
	Cervical vertebral instability. Malformation of the spinal cord, resulting in an inability to walk properly—"wobbler syndrome."
	Color mutant alopecia. Partial hair loss, dry coat, scaliness, and raised red spots on skin, combined with darkening of coat in patches.
	Enophthalmos. A sinking of the eyeball into the socket.
	Exocrine pancreatic insufficiency (EPI). Lack of pancreatic enzymes resulting in poor digestion, excessive hunger, weight loss, and diarrhea.
	Granulocytopathy. A defect in the body's ability to kill bacteria, causing stunted growth and recurring bacterial infection.
	Idiopathic megaesophagus. A disorder causing enlargement of the esophagus and leading to regurgitation of food and weight loss.

**Prospective owners should screen parents and previous litters.

Breed/Color	Defects and/or Disorders
	Persistent right aortic arch. A disorder of the esophagus that causes a puppy to regurgitate solid food. It may be surgically corrected.
	Portosystemic venous shunts. Abnormal blood vessel in abdomen carries blood around, rather than through, the liver. Results in a buildup of toxins, which causes poor growth, salivation, seizures, and death. Surgery can help.
	**Progressive retinal atrophy.* An inherited disorder producing progressive vision loss, ending in blindness.
Shar-Pei	*Amyloidosis.* The infiltration of the kidneys and liver with a starchy substance affecting kidney function and leading to kidney failure.
	Excessive facial skin folds, leading to infections and eye problems, often requiring surgery.
	Hiatal hernia, in which the stomach passes partially into the chest cavity through a hole in the esophagus.
	IgA deficiency. Immune system deficiency, resulting in upper and lower respiratory infections, inflammation of the upper ear canal (otitis external), and skin problems.
	Tracheal hypoplasia. An underdeveloped windpipe, leading to pneumonia.
Shepherds—see also "Large and Giant Breeds"	*Microphthalmos.* Failure of the eye globe to grow to normal size. May lead to blindness.
Australian shepherd	**Optic nerve colobomas.* Pits or holes in the optic disc. Vision may be impaired.
	**Retinal dysplasia.* Abnormal development of the retina, which may lead to blindness.
Belgian shepherd	*Epilepsy.* Seizures, convulsions.
	Lymphedema. Swelling and pitting of legs, usually hind legs, caused by abnormally developed lymph vessels.
	X-linked muscular dystrophy. Causes a stiff gait ("bunny hop"). Appears at 6–9 weeks of age.

**Prospective owners should screen parents and previous litters.

Breed/Color	Defects and/or Disorders
German shepherd	*Aortic stenosis.* A narrowing of the opening of the aortic valve, which obstructs the flow of blood, and can lead to fainting, collapse, and sudden death.
	**Cataracts,* present at birth, may not be visible until 2 months of age and may be inherited. Juvenile cataracts may develop up to 6 years of age and heredity is the usual cause. In puppies, both types of cataracts may spontaneously disappear.
	Cartilagenous exostosis. Overgrowths of cartilage from bones throughout the body.
	Cleft palate/cleft lip syndrome. Midline closing defect affecting the lips and hard palate of the mouth.
	Collagen disorder of the footpads. Soft, sore footpads.
	Cutaneous asthenia (Ehlers-Danlos syndrome). An abnormality of the connective tissue of the skin, resulting in loose, sagging skin, which tears easily.
	Deafness in one or both ears.
	Dermoid. A cyst on the eyelid. May affect one or both eyes.
	Diabetes insipidus. A metabolic disorder due to deficiency of a pituitary hormone, characterized by excessive thirst (polydipsia) and large volumes of dilute urine (polyuria).
	Diabetes mellitus. May surface as early as 2–6 months of age. Characterized by high blood sugar, excessive thirst (polydipsia) and urination (polyuria).
	Diaphragmatic hernias (peritoneopericardial and pleuroperitoneal). Abdominal contents enter the chest cavity through an abnormal hole in the diaphragm.
	Epilepsy. Seizures, convulsions.
	Exocrine pancreatic insufficiency (EPI). Lack of pancreatic enzymes resulting in poor digestion, excessive hunger, weight loss, and diarrhea.
	Factor VIII deficiency (hemophilia A). A hemorrhaging disorder.
	Glycogen storage disease. An enzyme deficiency resulting in hypoglycemia.
	Idiopathic megaesophagus. A disorder causing enlargement of the esophagus and leading to regurgitation and weight loss.

**Prospective owners should screen parents and previous litters.

Breed/Color	Defects and/or Disorders
	IgA deficiency. Immune system deficiency, resulting in upper and lower respiratory infections, inflammation of the upper ear canal (otitis external), and skin problems.
	Lumbosacral malarticulation—spinal malformation, causing pain, possible incontinence. Can be surgically corrected.
	Lymphedema. Swelling and pitting of legs, usually hind legs, caused by abnormally developed lymph vessels.
	Lysosomal storage diseases. Brain disorders caused by an inheritable deficiency of key enzymes.
	Mitral valve malformation. A malformation of the mitral valve in the left side of the heart, leading to heart murmur and eventual heart failure.
	**Optic nerve hypoplasia.* Underdevelopment of the optic nerve in one or both eyes.
	Patent ductus arteriosus. A condition in which a fetal blood vessel does not close at birth, causing a heart murmur and leading to heart failure.
	Peripheral vestibular disorders, causing head tilt, circling, and rolling at birth or shortly thereafter.
	Persistent right aortic arch. A disorder of the esophagus that causes a puppy to regurgitate solid food. It may be surgically corrected.
	Pituitary dwarfism. Caused by a deficiency of growth hormone. Results in lack of permanent teeth, retention of puppy coat, abnormal skeletal growth, and many other disorders.
Tervuren shepherd	*Epilepsy.* Seizures, convulsions.
	Lymphedema—see "German shepherd," above.
Shetland sheepdog	*Chondrodysplasia.* Dwarfism. Short front legs; paws turned sideways. Caused by poor cartilage and bone growth.
	Cleft palate/cleft lip syndrome. Midline closing defect affecting the lips and hard palate of the mouth.

**Prospective owners should screen parents and previous litters.

SOME COMMON CONGENITAL DEFECTS AND DISORDERS

Breed/Color	Defects and/or Disorders
Shetland sheepdog (cont'd)	** *Collie eye anomaly.* Multiple eye defects, including coloboma (pitting) of the optic disc.
	Cryptorchidism, in which neither, or only one, testicle descends.
	Deafness in one or both ears.
	Dermatomyositis. Inflammation of skin and muscles, probably caused by an abnormal immune system.
	Distichiasis. An extra row of eyelashes that may rub on the cornea.
	** *Hip dysplasia.* A deformity of the hip joint, leading to lameness. Onset usually occurs at about 5 months of age.
	Hypersensitivity to Ivermectin, a drug commonly used in prevention and treatment of heartworms.
	Microphthalmos. Failure of the eye globe to grow to normal size. May lead to blindness.
	** *Optic nerve colobomas.* Pits or holes in the optic disc. Vision may be impaired.
	Patent ductus arteriosus. A condition in which a fetal blood vessel does not close at birth, causing a heart murmur and leading to heart failure.
	Peripheral vestibular disorders, causing head tilt, circling, and rolling at birth or shortly thereafter.
	** *von Willebrand's disease. Factor VIII deficiency.* An inherited bleeding disorder.
Shiba inu	*Pseudohyperkalemia.* High level of potassium in red blood cells, causing falsely elevated readings on clotted blood samples.
Shih tzu—see also "Brachycephalic Breeds"	*Distichiasis.* An extra row of eyelashes that may rub on the cornea.
	** *Familial renal (kidney) disease,* which varies with individuals. May cause anorexia, lethargy, weight loss, anemia, excessive thirst (polydipsia) and urination (polyuria), and other problems.

**Prospective owners should screen parents and previous litters.

Breed/Color	Defects and/or Disorders
Siberian husky	**Cataracts,* present at birth, may not be visible until 2 months of age and may be inherited. Juvenile cataracts may develop up to 6 years of age and heredity is the usual cause. In puppies, both types of cataracts may spontaneously disappear.
	Laryngeal paralysis. Paralysis of the larynx, resulting in loud, difficult breathing.
Silky terrier	*Lysosomal storage diseases.* Brain disorders caused by an inheritable deficiency of key enzymes.
Skye terrier	*Laryngeal hypoplasia.* An incompletely developed larynx.
	Occipital dysplasia. Malformation of the occipital bone at the back and base of the skull, possibly exposing the cerebellum and brain stem to trauma.
Small and Toy Breeds: Bichon Frisé; Chihuahua; Jack Russell; Maltese; Papillon; Pekingese; Pomeranian; Schnauzer, miniature; Spaniels, King Charles and toy; Yorkshire terrier	*Cricopharyngeal achalasia.* Failure of the throat muscles to relax and permit food to pass through.
	Legg-Calvé-Perthes disease (aseptic necrosis). Collapse of bone and malformation of the hip joint, leading to arthritis. Onset at 5–9 months of age. May be corrected surgically.
	Neonatal hypoglycemia. Low blood sugar occurring during nursing age. Causes mental confusion, weakness, seizures, and/or coma.
	Patellar luxation. A dislocation of the kneecap, causing pain and lameness. Surgery may help.
	Tracheal collapse. Collapsed windpipe leading to coughing, bronchitis, and pneumonia.
Soft-coated Wheaten terrier	***Familial renal (kidney) disease,* varies with individuals. May cause anorexia, lethargy, weight loss, anemia, excessive thirst (polydipsia) and urination (polyuria), and other problems.
Spaniels	*Epilepsy.* Seizures, convulsions.

**Prospective owners should screen parents and previous litters.

Breed/Color	Defects and/or Disorders
Brittany spaniel	*Complement deficiency.* A deficiency of blood proteins.
Cavalier King Charles spaniel—see also "Small and Toy Breeds"	*Corneal dystrophy.* Corneal dullness, usually in both eyes.
	Microphthalmos. Failure of the eye globe to grow to normal size. May lead to blindness.
	**Retinal dysplasia.* Abnormal development of the retina, which may lead to blindness.
	Shoulder luxation. Dislocation of the shoulder joint, occurring at 3–4 months of age.
Cocker spaniel	*Anury.* The absence of one or more tail vertebrae.
	Brachury. An abnormally short tail.
	***Cataracts,* present at birth, may not be visible until 2 months of age and may be inherited. Juvenile cataracts may develop up to 6 years of age and heredity is the usual cause. In puppies, both types of cataracts may spontaneously disappear.
	Cleft palate/cleft lip syndrome. Midline closing defect affecting the lips and hard palate of the mouth.
	Cranioschisis. Soft spots in the skull.
	Cyclic neutropenia. Cyclic interruption in bone marrow production of white blood cells, leading to infections and fever.
	Deafness in one or both ears.
	Distichiasis. An extra row of eyelashes that may rub on the cornea.
	Ectropion. Eyelid turned outward, exposing mucous membranes covering the conjunctival lining, causing infection, ocular discharge, and swollen eyelids.
	***Familial renal (kidney) disease,* which varies with individuals. May cause anorexia, lethargy, weight loss, anemia, excessive thirst (polydipsia) and urination (polyuria), and other problems.

**Prospective owners should screen parents and previous litters.

Breed/Color	Defects and/or Disorders
	**Glaucoma. Usually develops after 1 year of age. Caused by increase in eyeball pressure and can lead to blindness.
	**Hip dysplasia. A deformity of the hip joint, leading to lameness. Onset usually occurs at about 5 months of age.
	Imperforate lacrimal punctum. Watering of the eye(s) due to improperly formed duct from the eye to the nose.
	Lysosomal storage diseases. Brain disorders caused by an inheritable deficiency of key enzymes.
	Neuronal degeneration. Nerve degeneration, causing tremors, shaky movements, and seizures at an early age.
	Occipital dysplasia. Malformation of the occipital bone at the back and base of the skull, possibly exposing the cerebellum and brain stem to trauma.
	Patent ductus arteriosus. A condition in which a fetal blood vessel does not close at birth, causing a heart murmur and leading to heart failure.
	Pulmonic stenosis. Narrowing or obstruction of artery leading from right ventricle of the heart to the pulmonary artery. May produce heart failure.
	**Retinal dysplasia. Abnormal development of the retina, which may lead to blindness.
	XX sex reversal, causing hermaphroditism and abnormal genital development.
American cocker spaniel	*Factor X deficiency.* A hemorrhaging disorder, causing stillbirth and early death.
	Phosphofructokinase deficiency. An enzyme deficiency.
English cocker spaniel	*Factor II deficiency.* Lack of a blood-clotting factor, leading to mild bleeding, lameness, and nosebleeds. Trauma or surgery may lead to life-threatening bleeding.
	Peripheral vestibular disorders, causing head tilt, circling, and rolling at birth or shortly thereafter.

**Prospective owners should screen parents and previous litters.

Breed/Color	Defects and/or Disorders
Japanese spaniel	*Lysosomal storage diseases.* Brain disorders caused by an inheritable deficiency in a key enzyme.
Springer spaniel	**Cataracts,* present at birth, may not be visible until 2 months of age and may be inherited. Juvenile cataracts may develop up to 6 years of age and heredity is the usual cause. In puppies, both types of cataracts may spontaneously disappear.
	Diabetes mellitus. May surface as early as 2–6 months of age. Characterized by high blood sugar, excessive thirst (polydipsia) and urination (polyuria).
	Factor XI deficiency. A deficiency of a clotting factor in the blood, causing minor bleeding. Trauma or surgery may produce major bleeding.
	**Glaucoma.* Usually develops after 1 year of age. Caused by an increase in eyeball pressure and can lead to blindness.
	Hypomyelination/dysmyelination. Reduced/abnormal insulating layer of myelin (material formed of protein and a lipid) around the central nervous system, causing rear limb weakness and difficulty walking.
	Persistent atrial standstill. A heart problem, requiring a pacemaker.
	Phosphofructokinase deficiency. An enzyme deficiency.
	**Retinal dysplasia.* Abnormal development of the retina, which may lead to blindness.
Sussex spaniel	**Retinal dysplasia—see "Springer spaniel," above.
Toy spaniel—see also "Small and Toy Breeds"	**Retinal dysplasia—see "Springer spaniel," above.
Spitz—see "Finnish spitz"	
Tibetan terrier	**Retinal dysplasia—see "Springer spaniel," above.
Toy breeds—see "Small and Toy Breeds"	
Vizsla	*Factor I deficiency.* Deficiency of a blood-clotting factor, which may cause bleeding.
Weimaraner	*Diaphragmatic hernias (peritoneopericardial and pleuroperitoneal).* Abdominal contents enter the chest cavity through an abnormal hole in the diaphragm.

**Prospective owners should screen parents and previous litters.

Breed/Color	Defects and/or Disorders
	Factor XI deficiency. A deficiency of a clotting factor in the blood causing minor bleeding. Trauma or surgery may produce major bleeding.
	Granulocytopathy. A defect in the body's ability to kill bacteria, causing stunted growth and recurring bacterial infections.
	Hypomyelination/dysmyelination. Reduced/abnormal layer of myelin (material formed of protein and a lipid) around the central nervous system, causing rear limb weakness and difficulty walking.
	Pituitary dwarfism. Caused by a deficiency of growth hormone. Results in lack of permanent teeth, retention of puppy coat, abnormal skeletal growth, and many other disorders.
	Spinal dystraphism. Spinal cord and vertebral defects.
	Tricuspid valve dysplasia. A malformation of the tricuspid valve of the right side of the heart. Leads to heart murmur and heart failure.
	Umbilical hernia. Swelling around the umbilicus (navel). May be surgically corrected.
	Ununited anconeal process. Elbow dysplasia. May occur in one or both front legs and may result in arthritis.
	XX sex reversal, causing hermaphroditism and abnormal genital development.
West Highland white terrier	*Copper-associated hepatopathy.* An overaccumulation of copper in the liver as dog ages, causing hepatitis and cirrhosis of the liver.
	Deafness in one or both ears.
	Diabetes mellitus. May surface as early as 2–6 months of age. Characterized by high blood sugar, excessive thirst (polydipsia) and urination (polyuria).
	Ectopic ureter. A misplacement of the tube or tubes that lead from the kidneys to the bladder. Females, especially, are often incontinent.
	***Epidermal dysplasia.* Familial skin defect resulting in warty growths.
	Ichthyosis. Dry, rough, thick, scaly skin, including footpads, which worsens with age.

**Prospective owners should screen parents and previous litters.

Breed/Color	Defects and/or Disorders
	Inguinal hernia. Hernia in the groin.
	Lysosomal storage diseases. Brain disorders caused by an inheritable deficiency of key enzymes.
	Pyruvate kinase deficiency. An enzyme deficiency causing premature red blood cell destruction and anemia.
Whippet	*Diabetes mellitus*—see "West Highland white terrier."
Wolfhounds—see "Irish wolfhounds" and "Russian wolfhounds"	
Yorkshire terrier—see also "Small and Toy Breeds"	*Cartilaginous exostosis*. Outgrowths of cartilage from bones throughout the body.
	Cryptorchidism, in which neither, or only one, testicle descends.
	Cystinuria. A defect in the kidneys, causing excessive cystine (an amino acid) in the urine, which leads to kidney and urinary-tract stones.
	Distichiasis. An extra row of eyelashes, which may rub on the cornea.
	Hydrocephalus. Accumulation of excess fluid in the brain and spinal cord, causing an enlarged head.
	Neonatal hypoglycemia. Low blood sugar occurring during nursing age. Causes mental confusion, weakness, seizures, and/or coma.
	Portosystemic venous shunts. Abnormal blood vessel in the abdomen carries blood around, rather than through, the liver. Results in a buildup of toxins, which causes poor growth, salivation, seizures, and death. Surgery can help.
	**Retinal dysplasia*. Abnormal development of the retina, which may lead to blindness.

**Prospective owners should screen parents and previous litters.

PROSPECTIVE OWNERS SHOULD BE AWARE THAT *MANY* BREEDS ARE SUBJECT TO THE FOLLOWING CONGENITAL DEFECTS AND/OR DISORDERS

Body wall	*Pectus excavation,* in which the breastbone protrudes into the chest cavity.
Bones and joints	*Polydactyly.* Extra toes.
	Premature closure of radius. Front leg bones grow unevenly, causing the ankle and foot to turn to one side.
	Premature closure of ulna. Outer, longer front leg bone fails to grow properly, causing bow legs.
Cardiovascular system	*Endocardial fibroelastosis.* The forming of fibrous tissue in parts of the heart lining.
Digestive system	*Abnormal dentition.* Abnormal tooth formation; retention of "baby" teeth; extra teeth; etc.
	Anorectal defects. Obstruction or stricture of the anus and/or rectum.
	Intestinal lymphangiectasia. Leakage of blood protein into intestinal tract through abnormal lymphatic vessels, leading to edema and hypoproteinemia.
Endocrine and metabolic systems	*Hypoadrenocorticism.* Congenital underdevelopment of the adrenal glands, causing early puppy death.
Eyes	*Entropion.* Inward-turning eyelid(s), usually lower.
Hematopoietic and lymphatic systems	*Factor VIII deficiency (hemophilia A).* A hemorrhaging disorder.
	Factor IX deficiency (hemophilia B). Females. Sex-linked bleeding disorder. Bleeding from umbilical cord, tail, feet, dew claws, and gums.
	von Willebrand's disease. An inherited bleeding disorder.
Reproductive system	*Os penis deformity.* Inability to retract penis into its sheath; may cause infection and damage.
	Pseudohermaphroditism. Occurs in both females and males in which the external genitalia do not match their actual gender.
	True hermaphrodite chimeras. Puppies that look like females, born with both ovarian and testicular tissues.

Respiratory system	*Bronchoesophageal fistula.* Improperly formed connection between throat and airways, allowing saliva and swallowed material to enter the lungs.
Urinary system	*Agenesis, or absence, of kidneys.* A fatal disorder, causing "fading puppy syndrome."
	Urethral anomalies. Malformations of the tube that takes urine from the bladder outside the body, usually causing frequent urination or incontinence.

Glossary:

Veterinary Medical Terms

and Canine

Diseases/Disorders

Mentioned in the Text

acute: Of sudden or rapid onset, as opposed to chronic

Addison's disease: An endocrine disease more common in female dogs. Causes appetite loss, lethargy, weakness, and vomiting. Diagnosed by a blood test, it can be easily treated.

adenoma: Benign tumor originating in glandular tissue

agenesis: Absence of an organ at birth

alopecia: Hair loss

analgesia: Loss of sensation of pain

anasarca: Fluid in limbs or under the skin (edema)

anemia: Low red-blood-cell count. Can be caused by blood loss or parasites. Also caused by immune-mediated diseases that destroy red blood cells (hemolytic anemia), or because bone marrow is not producing red blood cells (aplastic anemia).

anomaly: Deviation from the norm, usually congenital

anorexia: Loss of appetite

apnea: Complete cessation of breathing

arthritis: Joint inflammation

arthro-: Pertaining to joints

ascites: An accumulation of fluid in the abdominal cavity, causing swelling

aseptic: Free of disease organisms

atopy: Allergic reaction to inhaled allergens; usually appears as a skin problem

atrophy: Wasting away of an organ or tissue

aural: Pertaining to the ear

autoimmune disease: Disease characterized by the body's destruction of its own tissues

benign: A tumor or growth that is not malignant (cancerous)

bilateral: Occurring on both sides

biopsy: Removal of small piece of tissue for microscopic examination

bitch: A female dog

bloat: See gastric dilatation/volvulus (GDV).

brachycephalic breeds: Dogs with short, pushed-in noses and protruding eyes

canine tooth: Eye tooth, cuspid, fang. Third tooth from front middle in both upper and lower jaws.

carcinoma: A cancer that arises in the tissue that lines the skin and internal organs (epithelium)

cardio-: Pertaining to the heart

castration: Neutering of a male dog by surgical removal of the testicles

CAT (CT) scan (computerized axial tomography; computed tomography). A specialized imaging technique using X rays. A diagnostic procedure.

cataract: Opacity in the eye lens

chronic: An ongoing or recurring condition, as opposed to *acute*

clinical signs: Symptoms or signs that are able to be seen

colitis: Inflammation of the colon

congenital: A condition/disease/defect present at birth that may surface later in life. May or may not be hereditary.

conjunctivitis: Inflammation of the mucous membranes (conjunctival tissue) that line the eyes and eyelids

coprophagia: Stool eating

cornea: Clear outer eye covering

Cushing's syndrome: A common canine endocrine disease occurring usually in middle-to-old-aged dogs. Symptoms include increased appetite, thirst, urination; lethargy; muscle weakness; abdominal distension; hair loss; sexual dysfunction. Blood tests are used for diagnosis. May be caused by an adrenal tumor, which can be surgically removed. With proper treatment, the prognosis is fair to good.

cyanosis: Bluish discoloration of skin and mucous membranes, due to lack of oxygen in the blood

cyst: A fluid-filled sac

dehydration: A lack of water in body tissues. Symptoms include thirst, weakness, nausea, and skin with decreased elasticity.

diabetes insipidus: Rare metabolic disease due to deficiency of a pituitary hormone, causing increased thirst, urination

diabetes mellitus: High blood sugar due to insufficient production of insulin by the pancreas, or lack of insulin absorption by tissues/organs. Symptoms include increased thirst and urination, and weight loss.

diaphragm: Thin, membranous muscle separating the lung cavity from the abdominal cavity

DIC (disseminated intravascular coagulation): Bleeding disorder. Destruction of blood-clotting factors, leading to hemorrhage.

dilatation: Widening, expansion

dysplasia: An abnormal development of tissue or bone

dyspnea: Difficult breathing

dystocia: Difficult birth

edema: Excessive accumulation of fluid in body tissue, causing swelling

electrolytes: Ions, such as sodium and potassium, in the blood

embolus: Blood clot formed in one location that lodges elsewhere

encephalitis: Inflammation of the brain

encephalo-: Pertaining to the brain

enteritis: Intestinal inflammation

entero-: Pertaining to the intestines

EPI (exocrine pancreatic insufficiency): Common to young adult dogs. Symptoms include a ravenous appetite accompanied by weight loss, diarrhea, vomiting, and abdominal discomfort. Diagnosis by a number of tests; treatment is primarily dietary.

estrous cycle: Regularly occurring heat cycle of a female dog

estrus: The actual heat period

exocrine: A gland that secretes by means of a duct (e.g., sweat gland)

femur: Thigh bone

fibroma: A nonmalignant connective-tissue tumor

GDV (gastric dilatation/volvulus; "bloat"): Affects primarily large-breed dogs. Symptoms include frequent, ineffective attempts to vomit, followed by abdominal swelling. This is an emergency—see p. 50 for more about bloat.

gastro-: Pertaining to the stomach

glaucoma: Buildup of pressure in the eye

granuloma: A mass resulting from infection, irritation, or unknown cause

hematoma: Large blod clot

hepato-: Pertaining to the liver

hereditary: A disease or disorder present at birth that can be traced back to ancestors. May surface later in life.

hernia: Protrusion of an organ or tissue out of the body cavity in which it normally lies

hip dysplasia: Hereditary failure of hip joint to develop properly; usually leads to arthritis

hydration: Balance of water in the body

hydrothorax: Fluid around the lungs, also called pleural effusion

hyper-: An overproduction, as in hyperthyroidism

hypercalcemia: An abnormally high concentration of calcium in the blood

hyperplasia: Enlargement

HOD (hypertrophic osteodystrophy): Painful inflammatory disorder affecting the distal (bottom) end of the radius and ulna in large-breed, young, growing dogs. The cause is unknown, but may be related to over-nutrition and rapid growth.

hypo-: A deficiency or underproduction, as in hypothyroidism

hypoxia: A deficiency of oxygen in the tissues

IBD (inflammatory bowel diseases): Inflammation of the mucous membranes of the intestines, attributable to many causes. Symptoms include diarrhea, vomiting, and abdominal distress. Treatment consists of dietary management and some medications.

idiopathic: Of unknown cause

immune-mediated disease: Disease caused by inappropriate overreaction of immune system

incubation period: Time between exposure to a disease and the onset of symptoms

interdigital: Between the toes

intra-: Within

-itis: Inflammation of, as in *gastritis* (stomach inflammation)

jaundice: Yellow skin and mucous membranes, usually due to liver disease, pancreatic disease, or gallbladder disease

larynx: Opening of the trachea (windpipe) at the back of the throat

lesion: Disease, or damage-induced tissue abnormality

lipoma: Soft, slow-growing benign tumor of fat

MRI (magnetic resonance imaging): A new diagnostic image more sophisticated than CAT scans or X rays

malabsorption: A condition in which the absorption of ingested substances in the small intestine is reduced

malignancy/malignant: Cancer or tumor that can spread (metastasize) in the body

mastitis: Inflammation of the breast

metastasize: Spread to other parts of the body, as a cancer

metr-: Pertaining to the uterus

mycosis: Disease caused by a fungus

myo-: Pertaining to the muscles

myositis: Muscle inflammation

necrosis: Cell death

neoplasia: Abnormal cell growth

nephro-: Pertaining to the kidneys

neuro-: Pertaining to the nervous system

nocturnal: Occurring at night

ocular: Pertaining to the eye

-ology: The study of

oncology: The study of tumors

-opathy: Disease or malfunction of

opthalmo-: Pertaining to the eye

oral: Pertaining to the mouth

orthopedics: The study of bones and joints

-osis: A diseased condition, as in osteoporosis

otic; oto-: Pertaining to the ear

overiohysterectomy (OHE, "spay"): Neutering of a female dog by surgical removal of the ovaries and uterus

pancreat-: Pertaining to the pancreas

patella: Kneecap

perianal: Near or around the anus

perineal: To the left or right of the anus

peritonitis: Inflammation of membranes lining the abdominal cavity

pharynx: Back of the throat

pica: Eating of unnatural or harmful substances (e.g., stones)

pneumo-; pulmono-: Pertaining to the lungs

pneumothorax: Collapsed lung with air around it

poly-: Excessive

polyarthropathy: Nonspecific disorder affecting all joints

polycythemia: Excessive number of red blood cells

polydipsia: Increased, excessive thirst

polyuria: Increased, excessive urination

pruritus: Itching

psychogenic: Behavioral or mental in origin

pulmonary: Related to the lungs

pupil: Circular opening in the center of the iris, through which light enters the eye

purulent: Containing pus

pyo-: Pus in, as in *pyometra*

renal: Relating to the kidneys

retina: Light-sensitive layer in back of the eye

sarcoma: Malignant tumor of body-tissue cells

secreting/secretion: Discharging/discharge

shock: See Box, p. 53

squamous cell carcinoma: Malignant skin tumor in squamous cell layer (outermost layer) of the skin

stenosis: Narrowing of a tube or passageway, such as of the spinal cord

thoracic: Pertaining to the chest cavity

thrombosis: A condition produced by a blood clot

thrombus: A blood clot

toxic: Poisonous

trauma: Physical injury

unilateral: Occurring on one side

uremia: Buildup of poisons in the bloodstream due to kidney failure

vestibular: Pertaining to the organ controlling balance, in the middle ear and brain

vulva: Female external genitalia

Telephone Numbers and Addresses

American Animal Hospital Association (AAHA):

Veterinary hospital referral. Call 800-252-2242, or write: AAHA, PO Box 150899, Denver, CO 80215, or e-mail: www.healthypet.com. Important: Include the zip code of the area in which you need to find a hospital.

American Kennel Club (AKC)

Breeder referral representative service: information about breeders in all areas. Call 900-407-7877 ($.99 per minute)

Free Dog Buyer's Educational Packet. Call AKC Customer Service, 919-233-9767, or write: AKC Customer Service, 5580 Centerview Drive, Raleigh, NC 27606-3390

ASPCA National Animal Poison Control Center

800-548-2423; $30 consultation fee, payable by credit card. Open 24 hours, every day.

National Pesticide Telecommunications Network (NPTN)

800-858-7378. Free nonemergency information about pesticides, lawn-care, and gardening products. Open from 6:30 A.M. to 4:30 P.M., Pacific time, seven days a week, excluding holidays.

Index

About the Authors

Michael S. Garvey, D.V.M., is a diplomate, American College of Veterinary Internal Medicine (Internal Medicine), and diplomate, American College of Veterinary and Critical Care. He is director of the Elmer and Mamdouha Bobst Hospital at New York's prestigious Animal Medical Center, where he is also chairman of the Department of Emergency Medicine and Critical Care, and staff internist and criticalist. He frequently appears on radio and TV to discuss pet care.

Ann E. Hohenhaus, D.V.M., is a diplomate, American College of Veterinary Internal Medicine (Internal Medicine and Oncology). She is chairman of the Department of Medicine, head of the Donaldson-Atwood Cancer Clinic, and staff oncologist and internist at the Elmer and Mamdouha Bobst Hospital at the Animal Medical Center.

Katherine A. Houpt, V.M.D., Ph.D., is a diplomate, American College of Veterinary Behaviorists. She is a professor of veterinary physiology and the director of the Behavior Clinic, College of Veterinary Medicine, Cornell University.

John E. Pinckney, D.V.M., has been a director of the Miller-Clark Animal Hospital since 1976. The AAHA-affiliated hospital is one of the oldest exclusively small-animal practices in New York State and has been at its present site since 1903.

Melissa S. Wallace, D.V.M., is a diplomate, American College of Veterinary Internal Medicine (Internal Medicine). She is associate director, head of Renal Medicine Service, and staff internist at the Elmer and Mamdouha Bobst Hospital at the Animal Medical Center.

Elizabeth Randolph is an experienced pet writer. For many years she was pet-care columnist for *Family Circle* magazine. She is the author of ten pet books including *How to Be Your Cat's Best Friend, How to Help Your Puppy Grow Up to Be a Wonderful Dog,* and *Dog Training by Bash.* She has appeared on radio and TV talk shows to discuss pet-care topics.